Read what people are saying about

Fit for the Love of It!

"Between the lines is a strong sense of confidence.
Uche and Kary seem to know their advice applies to everyone
and this assurance is delightfully contagious"
~ Scott Mackay
President of Probe Research

"If you are looking for an intelligent and sensitive guide
to make your journey to fitness fun, then
Fit for the Love of It! will rock your world!"
~ Sean C. Stephenson MNLP, CH.t
Author of "*How YOUth Can Succeed*!"

"Kary and Uche are on fire. Spend ten minutes with this
dynamic duo and you will be blown away by their passion and
commitment to fitness.
Fit for the Love of It! is a big winner!"
~ Scott Taylor
The Winnipeg Free Press

"Kary and Uche have incredible enthusiasm
and passion for their mission."
~Tatiana Anderson
National Fitness Champion, author, and ESPN Co-host

Fit for the LOVE Of It!

Simple Strategies to Enjoy Fitness & Powerful Reasons to Get Started

Dr. Uche Odiatu and Kary Odiatu

First Edition

U.K.O. Enterprises

Canada

Published by U.K.O. Enterprises

For information contact: U.K.O. Enterprises, Suite 234, 162 – 2025 Corydon Ave., Winnipeg, Manitoba, Canada, R3P 0N5.

First Edition
Printed in Canada

Photography by Lisa Achtemichuk and Cary Castagna
Text design and typesetting by Kromar Printing

National Library of
Canadian Cataloguing in Publication Data

Odiatu, Uche
Fit for the love of it!: simple strategies to enjoy fitness and powerful reasons to get started.

Includes bibliographical references.
ISBN 0-9688258-1-8

1.   Physical fitness. 2. Health. I. Odiatu, Kary II. Title.

RA776.O34   2002   613.7   C2001-903807-0

In view of the complex, individual, and specific nature of health and fitness problems, this book is not intended to be a substitute for professional medical advice. Always seek the advice of a physician before beginning any diet or exercise program. The authors and publisher have used their very best efforts in preparing this book. They assume no responsibility for errors, inaccuracies, omissions, or any other inconsistencies herein. The completeness and accuracy of the information herein and the opinions stated are not guaranteed or warranted to produce specific results, and the strategies and advice contained herein may not be suitable for every person. The authors and publishers of this book expressly disclaim any responsibility for any loss, liability, or risk, personal or otherwise, that is incurred as a consequence, indirectly or directly, of the use and application of any of its contents.

ABOUT THE AUTHORS

Uche and Kary enjoy life to the fullest and look toward the future with excitement and anticipation. They currently reside in Canada where they are recognized as experts in the field of health and fitness.

Kary left a teaching career to pursue her dream of becoming a professional athlete. She attained her goal of professional status in the sport of women's fitness (IFBB Pro Division). She has represented Canada at international competitions in Greece, Poland, Australia, and the United States. Her tireless commitment to promoting fitness in her country is well known.

Uche was born in London, England. He began weaving fitness into his life at a young age when his family came to Canada. He represented Canada in an international bodybuilding competition in Madrid, Spain (1986) while attending university. Fourteen years later, he once again represented his country at the World Amateur Bodybuilding Championships in Warsaw, Poland (2000) while practicing dentistry full-time. He firmly believes that a balanced life brings peace of mind, which stems from a healthy lifestyle, exquisite relationships, and spiritual fitness.

Kary and Uche have combined their passion for learning and teaching by forming U.K.O. Enterprises– a company that is dedicated to empowering people with knowledge, motivation, and tools for enjoying lifelong fitness. Their message demystifies the subject and inspires immediate action. Together they have written articles for several publications in North America. They have also been featured in a series of lifestyle fitness commercials, which focused on topics from their book: *Fit for the LOVE of It!* The media frequently approaches Uche and Kary for their fresh outlook on fitness.

They especially enjoy their live presentations where they can interact with others and share their knowledge and energy. Financial institutions, sporting organizations, and learning institutions are only a few of the groups who have been inspired and entertained by their message. You can visit them on the Web at www.fitlove.com or contact them at fitlove@shaw.ca

DEDICATION

We would like to dedicate this book to you, the reader. By taking this next step in your evolution, you are staking your claim for health and fitness. It is our desire that you will take some of the concepts in *Fit for the Love of It!* and use them to create a healthier body and a balanced life.

**"Down deep in every soul is a hidden longing impulse and ambition to do something fine and enduring...
If you are willing, great things are possible for you."
~ Grenville Kleiser**

CONTENTS

Part One: $\mathbf{T}$**aking Action**

Part Two: $\mathbf{L}$**iving the Lifestyle**

Part Three: $\mathbf{C}$**reating Balance**

ACKNOWLEDGEMENTS

No book is written alone. We have been blessed to have many people in our corner. In our journey to date, there have been many special and unique individuals who have shared with us their time, energy, and knowledge.

We wish to express our love, respect, admiration, and gratitude to:

-Our families who have given us the gifts of unconditional love and support. You are the wind beneath our wings. Thank you for helping us fly: Sigrid, Ed, Grandpa & Grandma Larkin, Grandma Mary, Mrs. Street, Laurie, Bill, Mitchell, Mary, Peter, Nkechi, Goziem, Val, Chiedu, Carolyn, Justus, and Elias.
-Dr. Shannon Gadbois, a knowledgeable and caring professional whom we look up to and admire.
- Sue Mosebar, our talented editor who gave us a sense of urgency when we needed it the most.
-Deepak Chopra, a modern genius, incredible author, and health professional; he expanded our minds with his timeless insights into the human spirit.
-Tony Robbins and his entire Robbins Research Family for their super-charged commitment to sharing their tools for ultimate self-empowerment.
-Reggie Horne, our own peaceful warrior from Mesa, Arizona, who gave us the gift of friendship and insight.
-Elmer & Ruth Milbradt for role modeling future fitness and helping us with this chapter.
-Sean Stephenson for his expression of the limitless power of the human spirit.
-Dr. Brian Friesen, a modern renaissance man, who has been an incredible mentor and friend.
-Everyone at the Garden City Dental Center and the Southwood Dental Center.
-Scott Taylor, Winnipeg sports writer, for his encouragement and enthusiasm.
-Debbie McLaughlin, a likeminded traveler, for creating our cover design.
-Georgio Affonso for his friendship and technical support.
-Cary Castaga, our Winnipeg friend and likeminded traveller, who gives us daily affirmations on the incredible resiliency of the human spirit to dream and desire to become more.
-Leah and Wayne Scantlebury, who have given us insight into their family's daily plan for happiness.
-Maurice Brisebois, with whom we enjoy dreaming and networking.
-Dr. Kumar Gupta and family, who personify the words, life long learners.
-Terry Goodlad - for his excellent insights into the sports of fitness and bodybuilding.
-Lisa Achtemichuk and VJ Sharma, our likeminded travellers on this very cool journey.
-The Manitoba Amateur Bodybuilding Association for giving us the opportunity to expand our skills in motivation, leadership, organization, and administration. They have given us the chance to care about people's dreams.
-Kim Cyr and Linda Sango, Uche's hardworking dental assistants, who have put up with his insatiable desire to multitask.
-Neil DalRymple, of Assiniboine Fitness, who shares his passion for physical fitness with his gym members on a daily basis.
-Pete Monroe and family (RMC Group) for being excellent role models.
-Keith Penhall, a Winnipeg professor, who has been an awesome motivating spirit in our lives.

-Jeff Golfman, a Canadian entrepreneur, who reminds us continually about staying on course and seeing our vision through.

-Julie and Arthur Williams, an awesome couple, who manage to provide inspiration for all families to love, play, and work hard.

-Neil and Ann Matthies of Peak Performance for the exposure to the Phoenix seminar.

-Eileen Montroy for her beautiful insights into "Soul Psychology."

-Nancy Teghtmeyer and Lisa Zimmerman, Kary's childhood friends, who have been awesome examples of loyalty through thick and thin.

-Garry Bartlett and Doug Schneider, amazing photographers, who embody the concept of "working with passion."

-The International Federation of Bodybuilding (IFBB).

-B. Pat Burns for his dramatic coaching and insights on the power of intention.

-Uche's teachers at St. Paul High School, who provided an incredible environment for his early interest in global pursuits.

-Vernon Blake, a special Winnipeg man who passionately cares about his family.

-Tatiana Anderson, an incredible example of a person moving forward in life

-Debbie Karpenko, our Canadian Bodybuilding and Fitness Judging Chairperson, who consistently gives her best in moving the sport forward. Her ability to care and nurture her family's needs at the same time is exceptional.

-Harriet Rosenbaum and family, who are on their path, blending their individual talents and moving forward.

-The Neuman family, who are an inspiration for us in that they make family values number one in their daily lives.

-Teachers from Yellowquill and the Portage Collegiate Institute, Kary's early scholastic influence, who gave her a fantastic opportunity to learn.

-The Kreviazuk's, an amazing family in Winnipeg, who truly define the concept of togetherness and nurturing.

-All the fitness competitors and bodybuilders in Canada.

-Shelly and Bruce Paton, who give us unconditional friendship.

-Martin Zeilig, our friend, who gave us fantastic early support and encouragement to work on our message.

-Chris Guly, an incredibly gifted writer, who gives us encouragement and continually challenges us to be better.

-Carolyn Klassen, our travel agent, who tirelessly provides us with her best arrangement skills and personalizes her service.

-Joan Rivers, who provided Uche insight into the incredible tenacity and resiliency of the human spirit.

-Our amazing Canadian Bodybuilding Federation friends.

-All of our friends who fill our lives with love, light, and happiness!

FOREWORD

I first met Kary and Uche in 1998 when they spoke at Brandon University. Later, I was fortunate to hear them again when I invited them to participate in the first Body Image Network conference in Brandon in the fall of 2000. In the three years since our initial meeting, I have been drawn back to their message frequently. What connected for me upon first hearing them speak is evident here in the pages of this book.

There is no doubt that, for all of us, the September 11, 2001, terrorist attacks at New York's World Trade Center and the Pentagon in Washington represent a point of reference from which all our current thoughts are established. These catastrophic events serve to remind us that quality of life is more important than quantity, that optimism is essential in life, and that the power of determination in each ordinary person is significant. Perhaps we now see as a society what many of us individually have known all along; that is, powerful messages of determination, strength, and achievement are as effectively relayed through "every man" and every woman" as through famous people and spokespersons. Kary and Uche, although now having attained some measure of celebrity in their own right, are indeed ordinary people though with a shared gift for story-telling, expressed with an inordinate sense of optimism and a clear understanding of how to achieve goals.

Martin Seligman, psychologist and author of *Learned Optimism* has said that optimism is essential for life, health, and happiness. Through his research, he has identified human strengths that act as buffers against mental illness. Some of these are future-mindedness, optimism, interpersonal skill, work ethic, and perseverance. Seligman says; "much of the task of prevention in this new century will be to create a science of human strength whose mission will be to understand and learn how to foster these virtues in people." In general, optimism allows us to persevere in difficult times and to achieve particular goals. Having listened to Kary and Uche tell their stories and share their ideas on health and fitness, it struck me that they embody what Seligman describes as the optimist and that they are just the exemplars from which others can benefit and learn. Also, it does not surprise me that all of the human strengths mentioned above are characteristics that could readily be assigned to both of them.

When my husband and I first heard Kary and Uche speak, at the end of the talk, one of the tasks we were asked to perform was to list our personal goals of all forms. Now, three years later, we still talk about our lists and use them as the impetus for moving forward while focusing on enjoying life in the present. This is the kind of impact their message, and their method of delivering it, can have on those with whom they share it. In the pages of this book, I believe they have faithfully presented themselves and their energetic perspective. If a book can be said to be "active," then this is such a book. Kary and Uche give information, then encourage you to work with it through the various activities and tools they present throughout the book. There is tremendous motivational pull in this approach that is sure to engage readers.

As a university professor, when I talk to students about learning from what they read, I encourage them not just to be passive but also to reflect on and work with the material they are reading. As you read this book, you will find it a challenge not to be active. Through personal experiences and anecdotes, they share their perspective while inviting you to implement their recommendations. The hallmark of their public presentations is the way in which they use story-telling to illustrate their ideas. Through activities, tone of voice, and gesture, they encourage their audience to "buy in" and try what they suggest. I believe this book accurately and genuinely brings their presentation skills to life despite the change in mode of delivery.

As you learn from this book, I wish you success. As you explore your potential, I encourage you to be active– although my prodding is probably redundant given that Kary and Uche are right here with you to do it much more effectively.

Shannon Gadbois Ph.D.

Seligman, M.E.P. (1990). *Learned Optimism: How to Change Your Mind and Your Life*. New York: Simon and Schuster Inc.
Seligman, M.E.P., (1998). Building human strength: Psychology's forgotten message. *American Psychological Association Monitor, 29(1)*, January.

"You can't leave footprints in the
sands of time if you're sitting on your butt.
And who wants to leave buttprints
in the sands of time?"
~Bob Moawad

INTRODUCTION

CAUTION: This book does not contain a quick fix or a promise to be the one place where all your questions will be answered. Our purpose is to give you simple strategies to enjoy your fitness quest and powerful reasons to propel you into action – NOW.

There are many sources of information on fitness: the seemingly infinite internet, dozens of magazines, TV shows, personal/life coaches, thousands of books, countless health professionals, heck, maybe even your own mother! You've likely heard many times over how important fitness is to your life.

So let us ask: how many times do you have to hear the message before you act on it? Virtually all of us have heard the "hows" and the "whys." So why doesn't everyone look and feel the way he or she truly desires ?

The answer is simple: knowledge alone does not always inspire change! Each of us needs to go deeper. But, once we uncover our very own personal, strong, emotionally charged reasons, we are compelled to exercise consistently (and enjoy it), eat nutritious foods in the appropriate amounts (and savour them), create an amazing environment for the important people in our lives (and truly feel fulfilled), and enjoy getting older (without fear).

Are we being idealistic? No! We sincerely believe it is possible to accomplish this and so much more!

The most compelling reason for you may be found in this introduction. Or you may discover it on the very last page. You will know when it happens. Your pulse will quicken as you realize what you have to do and why you must take action at that moment. And when this happens, we want you to pause for a minute. For that exact moment will mark a turning point for you. It is a second chance for a renewed way of living.

Hey, everyone deserves a second chance!

This book, *Fit for the Love of It!*, is loaded with simple tips and well-researched strategies to be implemented immediately. A simple decision to incorporate any one of them is the starting point leading to the enjoyment of greater health for you and the people in your circle of influence. The time to make this very personal choice is NOW!

"The beginning is always today."
~Mary Wollstonecraft

Psychologists have reported that when someone is ready for something new, it often makes an appearance. There is a reason why you picked up this book. We know you are ready for a new way of looking at this important subject.

When the student is ready, the teacher will appear.

Whether you know it or not, you already have tremendous qualities inside of you. You may not be manifesting them at the level you want right now because of the all-too-common feelings of self-doubt, fear, guilt, physical pain, or lack of energy. These reasons work against you, holding you back from living the life you were meant to live.

Rest assured, as you read *Fit for the Love of It!*, you will realize you deserve more than what you've been giving yourself and much more than what you've been settling for. No matter what kind of health you and your loved ones currently have, there is a chance for you – maybe this is your second, third, even twentieth chance. But it's your chance to make new decisions and take action – life does not have to be the same again!

In the chapters "Attitude: Our Daily Bread" and "The Power of Intention," we reveal the awesome creative forces inside each and every one of us. There are powers all of us have at our disposal that only a small percentage of people ever put to use.

As we explain in the first chapter, "The Perfect Time Is Now," all it takes is one simple adjustment in your attitude towards fitness or health. We like to think of the analogy of a ship on a voyage across the ocean. The first day after a small adjustment in direction, nothing appears to be different. However, it isn't very long before that one-degree change has a dramatically noticeable effect. An entirely different port of call will be entered. The same is true of the small adjustments you'll decide to make regarding your nutrition program: the first time you eat the apple instead of the chocolate candy bar for a snack, you won't see any physical changes. But after a few weeks or months of better food choices, you will notice a difference in not only how you look but in how you feel.

Think of the messages in *Fit for the Love of It!* as a prescription for reinvention. By making changes in one area of your life, you'll experience the benefits in all other areas. Change is one of the most powerful forces in nature.

"The real voyage to discovery consists not in seeking new landscapes, but in having new eyes."
~Marcel Proust

Making health and fitness a priority in your life can be the first step toward enjoying a better quality of life: success in your fitness endeavours will spill over into all other areas of your life, especially your relationships.

But before you can begin to take good care of others, you must take care of yourself. The bottom line is that all of the relationships in your life reflect the most important one: the one you have with yourself. The only way to change your world is to change yourself first. You'll find empowering tools for your journey into this new lifestyle in the "Spiritual Fitness" chapter.

If you lead a stressful existence, paying little attention to your physical, emotional, or spiritual self, there will eventually be dire consequences. See the chapter "Creating Balance" for powerful reasons to pay attention to other areas, besides the physical, in your life.

The chapter "Set a Goal, Get a Goal" describes the disciplined effort of doing what you have to do when you have to do it. This chapter assists you in organizing and prioritizing your dreams. It is a call to ACTION.

"**To become aware of the possibility of
the search is to be onto something."**
~Walker Percy

In the Zen tradition, sages talk of the beginner's mind – the ability to have an open mind when you are looking at new information. Whenever we read, we have found that by asking the question, "How can this information serve me?" miracles can happen. This process is called *cognitive restructuring*. Just by reading highly charged material, changes may occur. You will find it hard not to pick up relevant information and start incorporating it into your daily schedule. You'll see, all this stuff sort of just sneaks up on you.

You will find that underlining and circling information can start the ball rolling. All of the quotes in the text have been carefully selected to enhance the material you are reading. If one hits home with you – write it down in your journal or hang it on your fridge. New facts will be impressed into your mind as you write in the margins of the book, highlight tips, and turn down the corners of the pages. Go ahead, mark it up – you paid for it!

We challenge you to not leave *Fit for* the *Love* of *It!* unfinished. Resting on your bookshelf, it will not accomplish anything. Putting to use the strategies that hit home for you will make a difference in your life. You'll find simple strategies for nutrition and shopping in the chapters "Food for Function" and "Shopping 101." We believe you'll make more than one adjustment. Some of the strategies may be new to you. Some you may have heard before. But, our prediction is that today may just be the day you'll say to yourself, "I'm ready; I'll give it a try."

We will provide you with an array of tools to assist you in your journey. We challenge you to be outrageous in your quest for a renewed way of living. Step out of the old box that may have confined you, and leap forward. Not only do you deserve it – it's your destiny!

Sport is often a good metaphor for life. In athletic events, before the game starts, winning teams have a game plan with key objectives in mind. Our challenge to you is to begin making your game plan for your health and fitness now. Write down three things that you want to change about your current lifestyle:

1.

2.

3.

With the preceding desires acknowledged and recorded, you have started a magical process. By placing your interests in writing, you have focused your attention and set time-tested forces in motion. Remember the words of Yul Brynner as the Pharaoh in Cecil DeMille's epic film *The Ten Commandments*? "As it is written, so let it be done!"

Whenever you pick up *Fit for the Love of It!*, come back to this place and reread your intentions. This *action* will reaffirm your resolve and help you become more aware of the information and strategies that will enable you to achieve your desires.

"The capacity to care is the thing that
gives life its deepest meaning
and significance."
~Pablo Casals

Part One:

Taking Action

"If you can conceive it and believe it
you can achieve it."
~Napoleon Hill

CHAPTER ONE

THE PERFECT TIME IS NOW
ဆ

There is no time like the present.

Think back to a time when you had a brilliant idea or felt motivated after an inspiring movie, a good book, or a conversation with a friend. A time when you promised yourself you would get started with your new exercise and sound nutrition program. But, something came up, and your good intentions were put on the backburner. You went about your regular routine, and the days, then weeks, and then months passed.

Knowing that regular exercise and healthy eating is good for you is not enough to make you do it. We are going to help you bridge the gap between "knowing" and "doing."

Intuitively, it doesn't feel right to do less than we know we're capable of – letting ourselves off the hook each day. We're left with that gnawing feeling that "there must be something more…"

When we postpone something we truly desire, the consequences are usually not felt the first day or even the second. But days of postponing add up to another average year. A lifetime of average years will be filled with: "I wish I had…" "If only I'd…" "Why didn't I…?" The years fly by quickly, and the excuses pile up layer upon layer. The resulting wall imprisons us. This prison of regret has a cruel and vindictive jailor – you.

Everyone has done it to some degree at one time or another. The spirit says yes, but the mind and body come up with excuses to wait! But, you know what? The Universe doesn't care about excuses or procrastination, only that talents went unused and things were left undone.

Life doesn't care how turbulent the ocean is,
it just wants you to bring your ship in.

THREE TRIBES, THREE CHOICES

Everyone has obstacles and different ways of dealing with them. Picture three prehistoric tribes wishing to relocate to better hunting grounds. During their search, they encounter a wide river. All three tribes know there is better hunting and living conditions on the other side of the river. Tribe one tackles the river head-on and does whatever it takes to make it over. Tribe two makes a few half-hearted attempts and finds many excuses why their efforts are not working, eventually talking themselves out of the need to cross. Tribe three sees the river, makes no attempt to cross, and sets up a permanent camp on the side they're already on.

We can all probably identify with one of the tribes mentioned above. Do you typically find excuses for not acting on your health and fitness goals or, like tribe number three, do you not even bother trying? Have you made a few intense efforts and then given up…. Saying, "I was never meant to have fitness in my life. Or have you been like tribe one? You had a vision of the kind of life you wanted for you and your family. And then you went after it and persevered until it was yours.

**"I expect to spend the rest of my life in the future so I want to be reasonably sure what kind of future it's going to be.
That is my reason for planning."
~Charles F. Kettering**

THE SEARCH FOR THE PERFECT PLAN

There are many books, magazines, workout machines, exercise programs, and theories about losing bodyfat and increasing fitness. But the simple truth is we don't need to read every book on the market (although we're thrilled you picked ours). In fact, changing our health forever is as simple as moving our bodies for a few more minutes each day and taking small steps toward better nutrition. In other words:

"Eat your vegetables and get outside to play."
~Laura Fraser, author of *Losing It*

It sounds too easy. There must be some catch. Life has become more complicated, right? Do I have to eat organic vegetables? Do I need to wash my vegetables with special detergent? Can they be frozen? How much should I eat? Can I put special sauce or reduced fat butter on them? Can I play first and eat after? Does it matter how hard I play or for how long? Can I play alone? What if fresh vegetables are expensive? The questions and excuses are endless, and by obsessively focusing on them, we indirectly postpone taking action. But the truth is…**THERE IS NO PERFECT ANSWER!** You know what? You just need to move forward. It's often better to just get started than to try and figure it all out. Otherwise, you may end up wasting an entire lifetime scratching your head because things weren't exactly right.

Information about health and fitness is abundant, but information alone does not equal success! Some of you are waiting for that perfect article or health tip before you take the plunge. Let us break the news to you: if you continue to wait for something outside yourself, it may never come.

You have to begin NOW to make those important health decisions. Yes, it is up to you. And yes, it's an inside job! You must start with the information you already know. Believe us, you know enough to get going. Take those first few steps on your own. They will take you forward. These early steps are the beginnings of an incredible journey.

The journey of a thousand miles begins with a single step.
Take a step forward, today.

Celebrate your decision to take action. Use the momentum of these early decisions to propel you a little further along your path. Like a ripple effect, these initial steps will affect the other areas in your life.

"I was sick and tired of waiting for the 'right time.'"
~Lisa Sefa

I was a thirty-something mother of three who had reached a point in my life when I felt disgusted with how I looked and what I was doing with my life. I saw an article about Uche and Kary in the local paper, and I knew I needed to talk to them. Their number was unlisted, but I remembered reading that Uche was a dentist. I located his office number and tried him at work. It took some ingenuity to get a busy dentist to take a phone call from a complete stranger, but I eventually managed to get him on the phone after a few tries. He could tell I meant business, and he promised that Kary would give me a call.

When I first met Kary, I told her I was ready to make some serious changes in my life. She found out how badly I wanted to make those changes when I told her that if Uche hadn't passed on my message, I was prepared to go to his office and pretend to be a patient! I was sick and tired of waiting for the "right time."

We started with some minor dietary changes and a beginner workout program. I felt so incredible making these small changes. I was so motivated that I gave up drinking and smoking too! Incredibly, eight months later, with Kary's guidance, I competed in a novice women's fitness competition and placed third!

DETERMINATION

Do you remember a specific time in your life when you put a massive amount of energy into getting something you really wanted? If you don't, then remember back to when you were a child and you wanted a special toy. Didn't you do whatever it took to get that toy? You bothered your parents daily, wrote letters to Santa, or prayed nightly? Remember leaving no stone unturned? The word procrastination wasn't in your vocabulary, and you did not believe in making excuses for not having it.

Can you imagine being able to harness that amount of determination and enthusiasm when you approach your health and fitness dreams? As you take that first step and begin to think about making a change in your life (which you are obviously doing right now!), then you must make a commitment and begin to act upon it TODAY!

Think of children learning to take their first steps—do they give up when they fall down? Of course not! What's more, everyone around them encourages them in their attempts. It may take months of trial and error, but all children eventually learn to walk.

Close your eyes and think of a step you could take right now that will move you toward a healthier lifestyle. Breathe deeply and picture how your life may change with this new step.

It often takes a crisis or tragedy to move people into action. All too often we hear of someone starting an exercise program after a quadruple bypass. Some people hit rock bottom before they come to the realization that their current practices aren't serving them; they have habits that aren't adding value to their lives.

JOURNAL ACTIVITY

Do you have any habits that do not serve you? Pick up that pen or pencil and begin writing in detail.

If you never take any action on these habits, how will your health suffer?

If you took action today, what positive changes could you expect?

Now, repeat the following phrase several times until you feel the power of the words and its meaning resonates throughout your entire body:

"I am only one, but I am one;
I can't do everything, but I can do something;
what I can do, I ought to, and by the grace of God, I will do."
~A prayer from *O, The Oprah Magazine.*

THE POWER OF CHOICE

The direction of our life's journey is carved out by the choices we make. A single decision made in a pivotal moment can determine the quality of the following years. The decision postponed or never made will also affect your life. To not think so is naïve.

Most of us have the power to choose the quality and quantity of the food we put in our bodies. We also have the power to put down the remote and go for a walk. No one forces us to eat the next doughnut or skip our Monday afternoon workout. No one. It's the choices you continue to make every day that keep you looking and feeling the way you do.

"If you are not willing to risk the unusual,
you will have to settle for the ordinary."
~Jim Rohn (author, and business philosopher)

MAKE IT A HABIT

Let us tell you a secret: anyone can have better fitness if it's made a daily ritual. What do we mean by a ritual? Here's an example: every day you probably do certain things at approximately the same time: brushing your teeth, eating, reading, and going to work. These actions have become mindless because you have made them a part of your daily ritual. At first it takes effort to make something a part of the daily ritual. We have to think about it and consciously do it. Yet in a surprisingly short amount of time (less than a month), it becomes a habit, changing our lives forever. (It has been said that it takes only 21 days to make a new activity a habit).

Be prepared to feel a little anxiety or discomfort when you make those early changes in your lifestyle. The first steps in a new direction are always a little shaky – a little hesitant. In the history of the planet, anyone who has decided to go in a different direction or break free from known boundaries has felt it. And that is where most people give up. They start to question themselves.

It is at those times that mental toughness and discipline must be in full force. Until you begin to feel and look better, the only thing that will keep you going in those early stages is your personal tenacity.

> **"I know if I got up, made it out the door and did a workout or completed a vigorous walk with our dogs, I would feel very good."**
> **~Uche**

There are occasions when I am not in the mindset of going to the gym or taking our dogs for a walk around the park. That's where I use my "mental gymnastics." In that fragile moment of indecision or procrastination, I take a deep breath and acknowledge that I am feeling tired or overwhelmed. I tell myself that it is okay for me to feel this way. But (and that is a really big BUT), I also tell myself there is another way I could be feeling.

I know if I got up, made it out the door, and did a workout or completed a vigorous walk with our dogs, I would feel very good. Focusing on the positive outcomes of renewed energy and satisfaction motivates me to take action. My next step? You guessed it. I get up and make the move toward the door.

SIX-PACK ACTION PLAN:

World-famous success coach Anthony Robbins in his best-selling book *Awaken the Giant Within,* reported that all successful people leave clues or pieces of evidence behind them. Study these clues and you can learn how to achieve your own results. So, if you are interested in or, dare we say, committed to having high levels of results and fulfillment in your health and fitness endeavours, seek people who are achieving the kind of results you're looking for.

We have listed six clues that we have discovered in our search for people who are making it happen. Please note – *waiting around* was not one of them!

If you wait until all the conditions in life are perfect you may never get the chance to act!

1. **Affirm**– Admit that outstanding health and fitness is absolutely necessary in your life. Tell yourself on a daily basis that you are going to take responsibility for the condition you are in.

2. **Plan**- Sit down with your day planner and schedule appointments for your fitness. Make it realistic and achievable, so you're not overwhelmed. Even one exercise session per week for the rest of your life is better than starting out too vigorously and then quitting after three weeks of intense daily two-hour sessions.

3. **Discipline**– Be your own coach and follow through with your self-promises. By being strict in the beginning with your new program, early momentum will help you keep your commitment. Early positive results will also set the tone for future successes. Do not tolerate laziness or procrastination. These behaviours are self-defeating, and they may indicate your reasons need to be stronger. We will discuss this later in our chapter on goal setting.

4. **Ritualize**- Find a time of day that works best for the new activity and stick with it. Studies have shown that doing a new activity at a scheduled time of day will help it become a permanent habit.

5. **Share**– The *Fit for the Love of It!* strategy is about creating powerful alliances with your loved ones. You will be more likely to keep your commitment if your significant other or close friends are in it with you.

6. **Celebrate!**- Reward yourself when you accomplish even the smallest goal. Don't wait until you have lost the entire 20 pounds before giving yourself permission to feel good. Get excited and reward yourself early. Smaller goals that get rewarded in the beginning give you a feeling of accomplishment and the sense that your goals are achievable. Every little step in the right direction, give yourself a pat on the back. Who cares if no one else does? If all of us waited for someone else to acknowledge that we were doing the right thing, we could be waiting for a very long time.

THE BOTTOM LINE

What is the bottom line? If you do not act immediately, you may never accomplish your dreams! The perfect time is now! When you feel that initial surge of passion and excitement, you need to focus energy into whatever you're excited about! Remember those feelings you had in the early stages of dating someone special? You know the ones we are talking about: meticulously planning the mood you want to create, anticipating great times, and living in the moment. We are asking you to take that same excitement and apply it to your desire for a healthier existence. When you have a desire for yourself or your family that is grand and far reaching, act on it right away.

Life can be incredible when you are living an active, fit lifestyle. Exceptional living is not just about accomplishment or striving for the things that money can buy. It includes the things money cannot buy – inner peace, health, vitality, and satisfying relationships.

SUGGESTED READING:

Celestine Prophesy by James Redfield
This is an excellent book that challenged the way we both looked at our lives. It inspired us to keep our eyes open to opportunities.

The Magic of Thinking Big by David Schwartz
This book may have been written over 40 years ago, but it has many timeless tips for creating a life by design.

"I have always been delighted at the prospect of a new day, a fresh try, one more start, with perhaps a bit of magic waiting somewhere behind the morning."
~J.B. Priestley

CHAPTER TWO

THE POWER OF INTENTION
ભ

**"Even if times are *so tough* that only one percent of the
population is fulfilling their dreams, with the United States population
at 250 million, that means 2,500,000
people will be fulfilling their dreams.
Certainly you can be one of 2,500,000."
~from *Wealth 101* by John Rogers and Peter McWilliams**

We believe "luck" and "chance" are overused words. For example: "I'm not sure how I won that race; I guess I was just lucky," or "Someday I'll get my chance." When life is lived on purpose, when there are clearly defined goals; anyone can see the opportunities and make things happen. This is the *power of intention* at work.

*"I feel luck can better be defined as
preparation meeting opportunity."
~Kary*

Some people might think it was coincidence I walked by a poster for a bodybuilding show when I was 24 years old. I went to the event that was advertised and decided right then and there I would compete the following year in the very same contest. This decision led to my fitness career, which led to worldwide travel and competition success.

When I look back to that day, I don't think of it as being lucky but rather an experience I was ready for. I was looking for something more. I feel luck can better be defined as preparation meeting opportunity.

**"I am a great believer in luck,
and I find the harder I work, the more I have of it."
~Stephen Leacock**

Instead of considering chance events as flukes or as fate, we challenge you to see yourself as having more control over the events in your life than you may have previously thought. Psychologist Carl Jung talked about chance events. He referred to coincidence as a bridge between science and spirit. In other words, there may be more than chance at play when you answer the phone and the person you were just thinking about happens to be on the other end.

Paul Pearsall, Ph.D., in *Making Miracles*, explained how events do not always happen separately from us, but rather, they are connected to our interpretations and actions. This can be an unsettling topic, but we urge you to suspend your current feelings and beliefs and read on.

> **"...becoming more conscious meant becoming more aware of all that was taking place within me and around me, how my inner world affected my outer world and vice versa. I realized that the more *awareness* I have, the more *choice* I have in how I create or respond to the circumstances of my life."**
> **~from *Living in the Light* by Shakti Gawain**

BRIDGE THE GAP

Focused attention has the power to narrow the gap between the things you want in life and achieving them. Focused attention has organizing ability. Focused attention has the ability to make things happen. You must know people who wanted something so badly, they worked at it day and night and got it. It's almost as if they said, "Move over world, I'm coming through."

You can apply this very effective tool to achieving more health for yourself. Or anything else for that matter. Simply put your attention on what you want and resolve to see it through to completion.

> *"I resolved to take better care of myself and show more gratitude for the good things in my life."*
> *~Uche*

Looking down at my left wrist one day, I noticed a small raised bump. It wasn't tender, and I couldn't remember seeing it before. It looked out of place as I flexed my wrist, but I shrugged it off as an enlarged tendon. A few months later, I noticed it was a little larger. I then remembered a friend of mine having a ganglion removed from her wrist ten years ago.

I thought: Would I need surgery? How long would I be off work? What if I couldn't practice dentistry again? I decided to take some action. I went to a medical doctor and had a formal diagnosis made. He palpated it first and then applied pressure with his thumbs. "It's a ganglion," he said. "You can have it surgically removed if it grows, or you can just leave it."

Several months went by, and I still hadn't taken any action. One day I listened to an audio book by Wayne Dyer, Ph.D., called Manifest Your Destiny. *He told the story of his wife having a growth on her thyroid gland. Their friend Dr. Deepak Chopra advised her to spend some time meditating on any meaning it may have for her. She spent some time over the next few months quietly sitting by herself thinking about the growth and its significance. It resolved mysteriously by her next medical exam.*

I decided to try this myself. I spent the next few weeks thinking of the significance of the small growth on my wrist. I resolved to take better care of myself and show more gratitude for the good things in my life. I also prayed for a complete resolution. A few weeks later, I took a close look at my wrist, and my ganglion had disappeared.

Consider this… On a sunny day, every child on the playground feels the warmth of the sun, 93,000,000 miles away. Yet a child with a magnifying glass can focus the sun's rays to "magically" burn a hole through a leaf. Similarly, you have the ability to tap into the amazing power of focus when you magnify the magical abilities of your mind. Anytime you take energy and concentrate it, you have the ability to make things happen.

Efforts that are spread too thin rarely achieve anything. There's no point in buying a new pair of runners and leaving them by the door waiting for the urge to strike you. Until you find reasons strong enough (see chapter Set a Goal, Get a Goal), nothing of significance will happen.

If your goal is to live a life of health and vitality, you'll need to go about it with focused effort. It's not just going to happen on its own. Focused effort means you will be actively looking for information about fitness. You'll be asking questions of people who already have bridged the gap between *wanting* and *doing*. With this kind of energy and enthusiasm, you'll find yourself in the right place at the right time for going across the bridge. Things will start happening in your favour to move you closer to whatever it is you want.

Did you know there is a physical part of your body (called the reticular activating system), which can be used to assist you in this process?

RETICULAR ACTIVATING SYSTEM

The reticular activating system is a network of neurons in the human brain that has specific functions. Maxwell Maltz, in *Psycho-Cybernetics*, explains how the reticular activating system acts like a heat-seeking missile whenever your interest is peaked.

For example, if you are becoming interested in your health, you may start noticing all the different types of food people eat. You may notice that there are three health-food stores on your drive home. Or if you are looking for a piece of home-gym equipment, you may notice more advertisements on television for fitness-related products. You may also notice more people engaged in fitness activities. You may say to yourself, "Why are there so many people out jogging these days?"

Of course, new health-food stores aren't popping up all over your route home - it's just that your focussed attention literally pulls things out of your environment and puts them at the forefront of your consciousness.

Remember when you were looking to buy a specific kind of car? And you spent all that time and energy on test-drives and then finally made the purchase? Remember after you bought it? It seemed like *everyone* was driving your make of car. You would see them everywhere. Well, it wasn't that a dealer had a huge sale. It was just that your consciousness was highly charged. Your reticular activating system was still on red alert.

This kind of *thought concentration* has many profound implications. It's like stoking a fire. Paulo Coelho, in *The Alchemist,* describes the phenomenon of how the Universe conspires to help anyone who focuses his or her intentions. Serendipitous occasions take place: you share a seat on the subway with someone who happens to be a personal trainer; you find out your company has begun to include physiotherapy as part of your benefits package. You may think it's luck or coincidence. But, NO – your intense focus and desire for health has attracted vehicles to take you closer to your goal.

**"To achieve what you want, be it health, success, great wealth,
or recognition, you must want it strongly enough,
with all of the might of your being, to achieve,
to possess, or to be healed."
~Howard Hill, from *Energizing the Twelve Powers of the Mind***

TAKE RESPONSIBILITY

Now is the perfect time to take matters into your own hands and avoid the "I wish I would have…" syndrome: I wish I would have spent more time with my family; I wish I would have spent more time taking care of my health; I wish I would have spent more time working out; I wish I would have eaten with sound nutrition in mind.

There are two things you can be sure of in life: excuses or results. Most people have a huge list of reasons why they have not achieved optimal health and vitality. But until they put their own attitudes on top of that list, they will continue to find excuses instead of the results they desire.

The perfect time is now. Remember the motto: "If it is to be, it is up to me." Take charge of your personal well-being. Take charge of your health. Take charge of your physical self. Repeat after us: "If it is to be, it is up to me. If it is to be, it is up to me. If it is to be, it is up to me!"

**"Life does not need to be changed. Only our intents and actions do."
~Swami Rama**

FIVE TOOLS OF INTENTION

1. Desire—Wanting something to take place in your life is the seed of creation; it is the beginning of everything. Author of *Manifest Your Destiny*, Wayne Dyer, Ph.D., reported that the Universe has no waste. Everything in our world has a reason for existing. So, every desire we have contains within it the necessary resources to make it a reality. If we dream of participating in a full marathon, then we are fully capable of doing so! We would not have the idea or inclination if it were not possible for us.

What is your desire for your health? Please write it down.

Why must this desire become a reality for you NOW?

2. Visualization—Robert J. Ringer, in *Million Dollar Habits*, depicted a positive correlation between what we visualize and the results we achieve. Having a clear mental image of our goals and dreams is vital to achieving them. Keeping your goals in mind and rehearsing the celebration of achievement are powerful tools that can keep you focussed as you move forward. Mary Lou Retton, 1984 USA Olympic gymnastic gold medallist, mentally rehearsed a perfect gymnastics routine thousands of times before she actually achieved her dream.

Close your eyes now and see yourself living the health and fitness lifestyle of your dreams. If it's a little unclear at this point, don't be disappointed. As you become more focused and make a stronger claim on it, your ability to visualize will improve.

3. Action—Once you make the decision to move toward health and vitality, it's extremely important to take immediate action to let the Universe know you're serious.

As soon as you say to yourself that enough is enough—that you're sick and tired of being sick and tired—that's the time to make a phone call to your doctor's office for a complete physical. That's the time to go to your kitchen and start clearing out all the junk food from the deepest, darkest depths of your cupboards. Concrete action steps done with conviction take you closer to your goals. And the only way to keep the fire of desire alive is to fan the flames with purposeful action! Jean-Jacques Rousseau once said: "To live is not merely to breathe, it is to act; it is to make use of our organs, senses, faculties..." There must be one action step you can do to show that you mean business.

What one thing can you do right now to make your fitness dreams a reality?

4. Reflection—If you can think of yourself as a creator in your life, take a moment to look at the conditions you've created in your life. After a moment of reflection, ask yourself where you need to make some adjustments. It may take spending a little time each day by yourself, away from the hustle and bustle, before you can begin to move forward.

It is very important to use a journal and record your thoughts, goals, dreams, and actions on a daily basis. Why not make at least a five-minute investment? After a few weeks, you'll know why you look and feel the way you do—you have written records!

**If you are serious about your quest for health,
then now is the time to purchase a notebook.**

**"A life worth living is worth recording!"
~Jim Rohn**

5. Persevere—We were playing a friendly game of "Gender Gap™" one night with some friends. One of the questions in this popular board game asked: "What is the most important character trait for success?" The answer wasn't your physical attractiveness, networking ability, or your choice of careers. It was GUMPTION! Successful people take the initiative to get going and have the perseverance to keep going—no matter what! They do not give up at the first sign of rejection or the first "No" or even the tenth "No"! They commit themselves to continual improvement and see each setback as a learning opportunity for future endeavours.

**"We all have dreams. But in order to make dreams into reality, it takes an awful lot of determination, dedication, self-discipline, and effort."
~Jesse Owens**

THE "BUT" BLUES

In the beginning, if you are far from your goal, it may take every ounce of energy you have to get the ball rolling. It will take some butt-breaking behaviour to get there. Yes, we said behaviour! Dr. Stephen Covey says, "It is impossible to talk yourself out of problems you have behaved your way into." It takes action.

The sad thing is most of us are challenged by "*but*-breaking" behaviour… "but I don't have time right now"; "…but I would like to start my program when I have enough money for a personal trainer"; "…but New Year's is just one month away"; "…but I have big bones"; "…but my spouse is very negative."

It is time to make the decision to end the "but blues" and move forward with your health and fitness goals. What are you going to do this very day that will make a difference for your future? If you don't do something different today, your tomorrow will be pretty much the same as yesterday. Days flow into weeks, months, then years, and life flies by.

A CALL TO ACTION

"Do the things that the average person doesn't want to do."
~Uche

YOU are the major factor in making a difference in the condition of your health today. You are capable of doing incredible things. If you don't believe us, think back to a specific time in your life when everything seemed like it was going wrong. If you are reading these words, you made it through that time and probably countless others.

We challenge you to use your remarkable gifts to make some adjustments. If you don't like something in your life, change it. If you don't like feeling tired in the evening when you're with your family, make some changes in your lifestyle. If you don't like the way you communicate with your significant other, try another approach. If you don't like the way you lounge around the house, start moving!

We know you have more powers than you may be aware of. Remember, you are remarkable! And because you have the power of choice, anything is possible. You can start by putting your powers to work for you RIGHT NOW.

JOURNAL ACTIVITY

First of all, state your intentions (e.g., I intend to create a body that will perform the way it was meant to or I intend to go for a 20-minute walk three times a week):

I intend to:

I intend to:

I intend to:

I intend to:

I intend to:

You have stated some clear intentions for yourself. This is a very powerful step to bridge the gap between what you want and getting it! Writing them down makes them appear more immediate and less abstract. This task will begin the process of bringing out powerful forces that may lay dormant inside you.

In our next chapter, we'll help you manifest your intentions through a powerful goal-setting process. As you work through the goal-setting exercises, remember to use the five tools of intention – DESIRE, VISUALIZE, ACT, REFLECT, and PERSEVERE. They will help you uncover your own power and move you toward the achievement of your dreams and desires.

Remember: THE PERFECT TIME IS NOW! Reading this book and taking ownership of your new knowledge is your call to action.

Vision + Knowledge + Action + Passion = SUCCESS!

SUGGESTED READING:

Awaken the Giant Within by Anthony Robbins
This is a powerful book full of useful ways to take immediate charge of your life. It is a passionate call to action.

CHAPTER THREE

SET A GOAL, GET A GOAL

&

"The best way to succeed in the future is to create it."
~Robin Sharma, author of *The Monk Who Sold His Ferrari*

"We wrote out another 100 goals,
feeling the pull of the future…"
~Uche and Kary

January 1, 1999. We are on the beach in front of the Surf and Sand Hotel in Laguna Beach, California. The waves are crashing on the beach, the sky is blue, and gulls are darting into the ocean, searching for fish. Not only is it the first day of a new year, it will soon be the first day of our marriage. We have made a pledge to each other that this will be the first day of a bond that will continue to grow stronger. We have purchased a blank journal—our couple's journal. In it we have written promises to each other that we will treasure for a lifetime.

We have also written down 100 goals and dreams for our future. At times, we felt goose bumps as the words flowed, filling the blank pages. It all felt so right and so powerful—our pact with the Universe. Seconds flowed into minutes; minutes flowed into hours…

One year later

January 1, 2000. We sit on the same beach and read the words we had written the previous year. We're amazed how many of our dreams had come true and how close we are to accomplishing many more. We don't stop there, though. That is not what we're about. We write another 100 goals, feeling the pull of the future…

"Nothing happens unless first a dream."
~ Carl Sandburg

Maybe right now is a good time to reinvent yourself. How? By charting your course and writing down your goals and dreams. This is the key to enlisting the assistance of powerful forces in the Universe.

We know what you're thinking: "Uche and Kary, tell me something different. I've heard it before…"

OK. So you've heard it before. And you're sitting around feeling a little disenchanted. The challenge you may be facing – even if you've experienced some success and have seen some of your dreams come true – is that you have stopped dreaming.

Be honest. Lately, have you sat down and done some real dreaming, leaving your limitations and circumstances out of the picture? Do you remember being a child with big, unlimited dreams for your life? When you were full of hope and felt that anything was possible. If you take action and follow the path to your dreams with that sense of infinite possibilities and boundless joy, you will be that much closer to their achievement.

In his book, *The Four Agreements*, Don Miguel Ruiz shares that living fully requires action. And that sitting in front of the television day after day denies life. This inactivity is an obstacle for you to express who you are. Begin taking charge today…

"Until one is committed, there is hesitancy, the chance to draw back— concerning all acts of initiative (and creation), there is one elementary truth that ignorance of which kills countless ideas and splendid plans: that the moment one definitely commits oneself, then Providence moves too. All sorts of things occur to help one that would never otherwise have occurred. A whole stream of events issues from the decision, raising in one's favour all manner of unforeseen incidents and meetings and material assistance, which no man could have dreamed would have come his way. Whatever you can do, or dream you can do, begin it. Boldness has genius, power, and magic in it. Begin it now."
~Goethe

WHAT ARE GOALS?

A goal is simply a dream with a deadline. Everyone has dreams, but not everyone sets the goals that make the dreams a reality. The process of goal setting is fundamental to success in every aspect of life. The benefits are plentiful. Being in pursuit of a goal adds life to your days. The journey becomes more enjoyable. Goals energize and enliven you. They are an essential part of a successful life and, above all, will get you leaping out of bed in the morning. Ask a successful person from any walk of life about the importance of goal setting.

Champions in every field consistently do the things that average people choose not to do—like setting specific goals. Just saying you want to get "in shape" is not a very powerful goal because it's too vague. You need to come up with a specific indicator of what someone in good shape would be able to do. For example, "I would like to see myself complete the 5km Father's Day Run in under one hour, three months from now."

> **"No wind favours him who has no destined port."**
> **~Michel de Montaigne**

BECOME A CHAMPION!

In life, we want good things to happen to us. The challenge is that we usually have only a vague idea of what we truly want. How are you supposed to shoot an arrow and hit a target that is not there? Can you imagine a sports team setting foot on a field without a game plan? Knowing the desired outcome is vital to getting anything and everything out of life.

Goal setting is the place to start. It signals what direction you want to go. It tells you where you are aiming. You also need to determine the level of your desire to get there. What kind of fuel do you have behind your intention? Low-grade fuel or rocket fuel?

You are ultimately responsible for your life. The only person on the planet that can put all this into action is you. It's up to you to stake a claim for what state your health will be in. Each of us has a power system that is built in – WILL POWER. Some of you are saying right now, "I don't have any will power." Rest assured, will power is not inherited; it's something that can be built and improved upon.

To this day, no scientist or philosopher has been able to estimate the power and strength of the human will. Why would you set limits on yours? History has shown many people who have made a big difference in their respective fields with little more than an intense desire. The founder of CNN, Ted Turner, was ridiculed when he first proposed a 24-hour news channel on television. CNN? They called it "The Chicken Noodle Network." Michael Jordan was cut from his high school basketball team. Fred Smith, the founder of Federal Express, was given a C when he was in business school for his overnight delivery system business plan.

> **"Many people live – whether physically, spiritually, or intellectually – in a very closed restricted circle of their potential. We all have huge reservoirs of life to draw upon of which we may never have dreamed."**
> **~William James, the Father of American Psychology**

IDENTIFYING YOUR FITNESS GOALS

Take your pen and write down three specific goals in the areas of health and fitness. For example, your ideal percentage of bodyfat, a strength goal (e.g., I will perform ten push-ups), a new sport you would like to try (e.g., rock climbing), or hours per week you would like to spend on fitness, your ideal weight, an activity you would love to do with your family, a target resting heart rate (say, 65 beats a minute), becoming a non-smoker, drinking eight glasses of water every day, walking one mile every day… you get the idea.

Write them down as if you already do the activity or have accomplished the feat. Begin with the words, "I am" or "I have." The idea is to train your mind to see yourself already achieving the goal. Did you know research has shown that the mind cannot tell the difference between an intensely imagined event and a real one? Remember Mary Lou Retton from the previous chapter on visualization?

Close your eyes for a minute and breathe deeply. Picture all the wonderful health and fitness attributes you want for yourself. Once you feel certain, begin writing quickly.

> **" If I shoot at the sun, I may hit a star"**
> **~P.T. Barnum**

1.

2.

3.

Now, beside each of your goals, write a deadline for its achievement. If you only have goals that will take longer than one year to accomplish, then you need to come up with some short-term, smaller goals you can accomplish within the next year. It is these smaller accomplishments that will lead you daily toward the long-term goals. It is best to have short-term and long-term goals to keep your motivation up.

You can't get ahead with inactivity. Movement is vital to attainment.
Focused action toward a goal
makes things happen.

BENEFITS AND REASONS

Write one paragraph for each goal describing in detail what the benefits will be. These are the reasons. Reasons are the power behind the dream. Don't worry about how it will happen at this point. The key is to anchor strong and empowering reasons that will pull you forward.

Uche & Kary Odiatu

If your goal is to run in the Boston Marathon and you live in Moose Jaw, Canada, it's more important to know *why* you want to run than *how* you're going to get there. As long as your *why* is powerful enough, the *how* will appear.

As you're setting your goals, it is important to act as if failure is impossible or not even an issue. Before you start this next part, we ask that you put yourself in a state of total certainty. Remember when you were a child and it was the night before your birthday or the night before Christmas? You could barely sleep because you knew that the next day would be filled with great joy.

If you have some music that really motivates you, use it to heighten your state of total certainty. With your music in the background, breathe deeply and really feel all that bound-up energy in your body. Once you have captured these emotions, we ask that you begin writing down the reasons behind each of those three goals you wrote earlier.

1.

2.

3.

"The people who get on in this world are the people
who get up and look for the circumstances they
want, and if they can't find them, make them."
~ George Bernard Shaw

EXCUSES

Write down one excuse that has prevented you from acting on each one of your goals stated previously. It will put them into perspective maybe for the first time. You may even feel pretty silly writing them down at this point after you have written all the powerful reasons why your dreams must come true. You may even start to think of how those reasons or excuses have affected your life. Don't get discouraged. Remember, it has been said that awareness alone can start the process of change.

1.

2.

3.

"Life is full of excuses to feel pain, excuses not to live,
excuses, excuses, excuses."
~Erica Jong

PAINFUL CONSEQUENCES

Write down a paragraph for each of your goals outlining the results of not following through. Dig deep and expose in detail any consequences you will experience if you do not change your current habits and start to live your fitness plan. What will you think of yourself if you do not make it happen? What could you lose if you do not begin to take care of your physical self?

1.

2.

3.

TAKE ACTION

At this point, we know you are aware of the importance of setting goals. It is simple and easy to apply these techniques to your quest for fitness. We hope we have convinced you how easy it is. We have guided you through the entire process that champions use.

Did you take the required action and write down your goals? Just reading this chapter will not get you closer to looking and feeling good. If you completed all the exercises, congratulations: you are well on your way. If you didn't, why wouldn't you take advantage of the magic of goal setting? Seize this moment to go back and do the exercises. Even if you wrote only one goal, it could be the one that kick starts your fitness quest. Don't settle for anything less than you deserve. Life is too short to just get by with average health expectations. One poet wrote poignant truths about the pain of regret:

> I bargained with Life for a penny,
> And Life would pay no more,
> However I begged at evening
> When I counted my scanty store.
> For Life is a just employer,
> He gives you what you ask,
> But once you have set the wages,
> Why, you must bear the task.
> I worked for a menial's hire,
> Only to learn, dismayed,
> That any wage I had asked of Life,
> Life would have willingly paid.

We all deserve to enjoy excellent health and vitality. By simply defining what we want, asking for it, and then going about it with a focused plan, the ball can be set in motion for its achievement.

> "There is nothing like a dream to create the future.
> Utopia today, flesh and blood tomorrow."
> ~Victor Hugo

SUGGESTED READING:

The Magic of Getting What You Want by David J. Schwartz
This book provides a step-by-step method for putting your dreams into action. Its strategies can be used for any of your desires - excellent health, a fulfilling career, or a rewarding family life.

"Happiness does not come from doing easy work but from the afterglow of satisfaction that comes after the achievement of a difficult task that demanded our best."
~Theodore I. Rubin

Part Two:

Living the Lifestyle

"I don't think anything is unrealistic if you believe you can do it. I think if you are determined enough and willing to pay the price, you can get it done."
~Mike Ditka

CHAPTER FOUR

ATTITUDE: Our Daily Bread!
&

"Keep my words positive: words become my behaviours.
Keep my behaviours positive: behaviours become my habits.
Keep my habits positive: habits become my values.
Keep my values positive: values become my destiny.
There is no dress rehearsal. This is one day in your life."
~Mahatma Gandhi

"Everything can be taken from a person but one thing:
to choose one's attitude in any given set of circumstances—
to choose one's way."
~Viktor Frankl (concentration camp survivor)

Attitude is defined in the Oxford dictionary as: "A person's way of interpreting or reacting to his or her world." As much as our attitudes are looked on as individual commodities, we have noticed that our families also play a significant role in the development of our attitudes. And our early role models definitely played a part in shaping the attitudes we have toward health and fitness.

If you grew up in an active household where physical fitness was a priority, you probably find it easy to include some form of fitness in your life. If physical fitness was not a part of your upbringing, you may find it challenging to accept it into your present schedule. Your attitude toward fitness may be that it is time-consuming, boring, and painful, and thus, you will not make it a priority. The good news is that at any age, you can choose to have an **updated attitude**.

This chapter explores how your attitude affects everything in your life. Yet like the set of a sail, you can adjust your attitude to take you to a new destination—a place where you will enjoy an energetic, flexible, and powerful body.

DID YOU KNOW?

Being an optimist could be one of the best things you can do for your physical health. A study at the Mayo Clinic found that pessimists had a 19% increased mortality rate over the optimists. But there is hope! There are experts that say optimism is a skill that can be learned.

STINKING THINKING!

Did you know each of us has approximately 50,000 thoughts a day? Our senses are receiving information all the time; not a second goes by without having a single thought! Picture your mind as a factory producing thousands of thoughts every day. The conveyor belt keeps moving a thought continuously down past the viewing area to the collection bin. Sadly, research has shown that approximately 80% of thoughts are negative or self-deprecating. "I am destined to stay out of shape." "I hate the way I look." "I am not good at sports." You get the picture? And like a factory that produces poor quality goods, there are consequences.

Deepak Chopra, M.D. (*Magical Mind, Magical Body* audiocassette series) reported that every thought has a physiological effect on our bodies. Every cell in your body is eavesdropping on your internal (what we say to ourselves in our minds) and external (the things we say out loud) dialogue. Just by thinking about a negative incident from your past, you not only relive it in your mind, your body will experience a response as well. You may remember a nasty argument you had with a loved one or friend. Every time you remember the incident, you indirectly affect your body because the body does not distinguish a real event from a memory. Can you imagine the impact that years of replaying old scenarios will have on your entire body?

"It was not that I had intended to look and feel unhealthy.
It was just my attitude of expecting less for myself…"
~Uche

When I graduated from dental school and entered private practice, I thought I would have to scale down my expectations for my fitness level. I felt that a busy dentist would not have the time to spend in the gym like I did as a student. I began to exercise a little less and eat a little more. And over an eight-year period, my fitness level decreased dramatically.

This one time competitive athlete now had love handles. I didn't do any aerobic exercise, so I would become winded with the slightest exertion. My pant size grew, and I would make excuses for wearing oversized clothing: "Designer wear is supposed to be loose."

The sad part was I knew deep inside that this was not how I had planned on feeling. I knew I did not like the way I looked. But I still had the belief that it was impossible to have above-average fitness as a busy professional.

I was now living out the consequences of my belief system. It was not that I had intended to look and feel unhealthy. It was just that my attitude of expecting less for myself because of a preconceived notion had penetrated my everyday thinking and behaviour.

**"I always felt that my greatest asset was not my
physical ability; it was my mental ability."
~Bruce Jenner (Olympic Decathlon Champion)**

WORRY AND YOUR BODY

**"Worry is a sustained form of fear
caused by indecision."
~Brian Tracy**

Like negative thinking, worry can also take its toll on your body. Where do you think the phrase: "I worried myself sick" came from? Many people dump toxic waste into their bodies by way of their thoughts.

In the Phoenix Seminar program, Brian Tracy, a peak human performance specialist, did some intriguing research about worrying. He said that only 8% of all your worries are substantial and that only half of these worries, about 4%, are in your control! In other words, 96% of our worries are needless – you cannot change the past and petty issues are a waste of your mental power. Worry, which is really just "stewing without doing," says Mark Victor Hanson (coauthor of *Chicken Soup for the Soul*), will ultimately drain the mind and body of energy.

> "Therefore do not worry about tomorrow,
> for tomorrow will worry about itself.
> Each day has enough trouble of its own."
> ~Matthew 6:34 (NIV)

WORRY BUSTER

It is almost impossible to worry about something you are actively working on. In other words, TAKE ACTION! The first step may be as simple as writing down some of your main worries and deciding how you can approach them.

> "Let our advance worrying become advance thinking and planning."
> ~Winston Churchill

JOURNAL ACTIVITY

Write down just one of your health worries:

Now, write down three actions steps you can begin doing today to TAKE CHARGE of this important area.

1.

2.

3.

> "You are what your deep driving desire is,
> As your desire is, so is your will,
> As your will is, so is your deed,
> As your deed is, so is your destiny."
> ~Brihadaranyaka Upanishad IV, 4.5

THE HUMAN MIND

We know how easy it is to let our minds wander and dwell on negative thoughts. It is easy to give up control and allow your thoughts to drift from worry to fear. Being afraid can lead to being immobilized. Progress can begin to look impossible. The mechanism that changes the set of your sail can become rusted and antiquated.

We have to take care of our minds like any other vital system in our bodies. If we want to strengthen our muscles, we must progressively add resistance. Similarly, the mind can do incredible things if challenged. By using mind management, we can achieve life management and attract anything we want in our lives. Does this point intrigue you? If it does, then read on.

"One way to get high blood pressure is to go mountain climbing over molehills."
~Earl Wilson

THREE STEPS TO MIND MANAGEMENT

1. Be more conscious of your daily thoughts and how they may be affecting your actions. Whenever you become aware of a repetitive negative thought pattern, ask yourself: "Are these thoughts taking me closer toward what I want or further away?"

2. Be conscious of who you are spending time with (see the chapter – Who Is in Your Flock) for people also can affect your thinking. It is naïve to think they don't.

3. Begin reading books about great people who achieved considerable accomplishments against seemingly insurmountable odds. Reading increases your exposure to other people's experiences, and it will expand your consciousness.

"A man's mind stretched to a new idea never goes back to its original dimensions."
~Oliver Wendell Holmes

"Whenever I need a boost, feel overwhelmed or immobilized,
I go to one of the big bookstores in our city and look
through the biography section for inspiration."
~Uche

As I search through the shelves, one or two books will draw my attention, and I usually find a message or some inspiration within the pages. (The only challenge is that I will also purchase four or five books on sale at the same time.) The answers to virtually all the questions in the world can be found in books. Jim Rohn, one of our favourite philosophers, calls the process tapping the treasure chest.

DID YOU KNOW?
66% of adults do not read another
non-fiction book after high school?
(From Self-Development Guru, Brian Tracy's Phoenix Seminar Program)

A WINNER'S ATTITUDE

Having an achiever's attitude is akin to having mastery over your mind. Throughout history, it has been seen that peoples' thoughts play a large role in the quality of their lives. Milton in his book, *Paradise Lost*, wrote, "The mind is its own place, and in itself can make a Heaven of Hell, a Hell of Heaven." Shakespeare once said, "There is nothing good or bad, but thinking makes it so." Emerson reported, "Great men are those who see that thoughts rule the world." Do we need to go on? Okay, one more. Proverbs 23.7, "As a man thinketh in his heart, so he is."

The more you think about fitness, the more likely you will recognize things in your environment which will take you closer to your goal. (Remember your reticular activating system? It will zone in on anything in your environment that supports your conscious thoughts). The desire to get in shape will lead you in the direction of achieving that goal. The stronger the desire, the more thought you will put into it.

"The greatest discovery of our generation is that human beings, by
changing the inner attitudes of their minds,
can change the outer aspects of their lives."
~William James

If you have any kind of desire to do anything in your life, know it is possible for you! (Obviously, at this time it is a deep desire for more health in your life.) By focussing your thoughts in a positive way toward your desire for more energy and vigour, you will start to attract the people, things, and events needed to make it happen.

> **"I was overwhelmed with the knowledge that everyone has the ability to create his or her own reality: our attitude is our choice!"**
> **~Kary**

World-renowned author Wayne W. Dyer reported that the Universe does not have any waste. Every desire we have for ourselves is perfect. We have within us everything we need to bring about what we desire.

I had this concept demonstrated to me at a conference in Orlando, Florida when I was told to get a partner for an upcoming exercise. I felt a tap on my back and when I turned around, I saw a small man in a wheelchair who obviously had some kind of physical challenge. He was about the height of a three year old and had some physical deformities and a huge grin! He introduced himself and asked if I would be his partner. I felt a surge of sympathy and replied, "Of course!"

In the exercise, we were to share our reasons why we were not having success with one area of our lives. I was dumbfounded when my partner spoke. I had immediately thought his reasons would centre on his disabilities and his wheelchair. To my surprise, he began talking about the book he was writing and how he needed to commit to getting it done. I found out that he was a much-sought-after motivational speaker who had met and spoken with Bill Clinton at the White House!

When I had my turn, I brought up my reasons for not having the abundant life I dreamed of: my partner slapped a wad of bills in my hand and said, "It's not that scary, babe!"

I was overwhelmed with the knowledge that everyone has the ability to create his or her own reality: our attitude is our choice!

> **"People are just about as happy as they make up their minds to be."**
> **~Abraham Lincoln**

GUMPTION

The more we learn about people who have accomplished their goals, the more we realize that success is not based purely on physical attributes, social contacts, or intelligence. Remember the word GUMPTION we talked about earlier? It is defined as an attitude of *make it happen* and endless initiative with a sense of purpose!

We read the story of Regis Philbin in his book, *I'm Only One Man*. The feisty fellow grew up in the Bronx in a modest house where he lived with his parents, an Italian grandmother, an uncle, and a great aunt. After his stint in the Navy, he packed up and went to California because he had a dream of being a broadcaster. At his first job, he worked as a stagehand – hauling furniture and setting up props for TV shows! Even though he wasn't broadcasting, he kept his dream alive by working in the industry. He wanted to get noticed; he posted critiques, which poked fun at the shows he worked for. Someone noticed his GUMPTION! They liked his writing style and offered him a whopping $5.00 per week to do some writing and producing for a sports show.

One day he got an opportunity – he filled in for a broadcaster who was hung-over and didn't show up. "Here was my chance. I had dreamed about it for years. My knees were actually knocking. My heart began to beat so fast I thought I would have a heart attack on the set."

When he was done, he knew he wanted more, but it was not to be in this job. He eventually got a job with a radio station in San Diego, where he worked for years building up his reputation and eventually landed his first talk show. The rest is history…

"Nothing in the world can take the place of perseverance.
Talent will not;
nothing is more common than unsuccessful men with talent.
Genius will not; unrewarded genius is almost a proverb.
Persistence and determination alone are omnipotent."
~Calvin Coolidge

PEOPLE WHO OVERCAME THE ODDS

- Abraham Lincoln became president of the United States with a history of numerous election defeats, personal bankruptcy, and many family tragedies.

- Oprah Winfrey has become one of the most influential people in North America. She was raised in an abusive environment and she had a stillborn baby during her teen years.
- Sam Walton, legendary founder of Wal-Mart, grew up during the depression in a family divided by divorce.

FIVE ACTION STEPS

1. For one day, completely be in tune with your thoughts. Pay attention to everything you're thinking or saying to yourself. Whenever an undesirable thought or picture enters your mind, aim to immediately substitute it with one that is pleasant. Think of your mind like a VCR where your every thought is played out. Unless you take control of what's on the screen, you'll forever be watching images that make you feel lousy. Would you rent a movie and watch it over and over if you didn't enjoy it the first time?

2. If you are ever feeling down, instead of reaching for coffee or the phone or turning on the television, try some physical activity. When you exercise, your blood gets pumping, and your respiration increases. In Chapter 10 – Move It or Lose It, we explain the endorphins that are released when you exercise. These endorphins are known as the "feel-good hormones." One of our favourite phrases is, "Motion creates emotion."

3. Have an arsenal of positive images for your personal inner reference library. Call this your positive emotional bank account. For example, recall:

   - The time you won an athletic award
   - Any special events or occasions with your family
   - A job promotion or special task done well
   - The completion of an important project

4. Make a list of positive self-affirmations and read them! Carry them with you. It may sound corny, but everyone needs to be reminded how special they are.

5. Try listening to audio books or beautiful music while driving. We often listen to audiotapes during long road trips. It's one of our favourite ways to spend less time on unproductive thinking. (We don't recommend listening to meditation tapes while you are on the road!)

"The longer I live, the more I realize the impact of attitude on life. Attitude, to me, is more important than facts. It is more important than the past, than education, than money, than circumstances, than failures, than successes, than what other people think or say or do. It is more important than appearance, giftedness, or skill. It will make or break a company... a church... a home. The remarkable thing is we have a choice every day regarding the attitude we will embrace for that day. We cannot change the inevitable. The only thing we can do is play on the one string we have, and that is our attitude... I am convinced that life is 10% what happens to me, and 90% how I react to it. And so it is with you...we are in charge of our Attitudes."
~Charles Swindoll

A NEW WAY OF THINKING

Remember when we mentioned the concept of a one-degree change in attitude? One little adjustment will not appear to make a great difference the first few hours; however, a few weeks later, an entirely new port will be reached!

JOURNAL ACTIVITY

Is there a small adjustment you could make in the set of your sail when it comes to health and fitness? Please write it down.

Where will you be one year from now – what kind of life will you be living if you commit to that one small adjustment?

"I'm starting with the man in the mirror. I'm asking him to change his ways. And no message could have been any clearer – if you wanna make the world a better place, take a look at yourself, and then make a change."
~Siedah Garrett and Glen Ballard
(From the song: "Man in the Mirror" by Michael Jackson)

SUGGESTED READING:

Psycho-Cybernetics by Maxwell Maltz.
This book is a classic in personal development. Even though it was published in 1960, it contains many timeless strategies for making positive changes in your life.

Chicken Soup for the Soul by Jack Canfield and Mark Victor Hansen.
We had the pleasure of meeting the two men who put this collection of 101 stories together. If you desire some humour, wisdom and hope, give this book a read.

How YOUth Can Succeed! by Sean Stephenson.
This book is excellent for young people. This twenty-something author has a special message that will inspire and move its readers into taking action.

Time
~An essay by Arnold Bennett

Time is the inexplicable raw material of everything. With it, all is possible; without it, nothing. The supply of time is truly a daily miracle; an affair genuinely astonishing when one examines it. You wake up in the morning, and lo! Your purse is magically filled with 24 hours of the unmanufactured tissue of the universe of your life! It is yours... no one ever receives either more or less than you receive.

You have to live on this 24 hours of daily time. Out of it you have to spin health, pleasure, money, content, respect, and the evolution of your immortal soul. Its right use, its most effective use, is a matter of the highest urgency and the most thrilling actuality. If one cannot arrange that an income of 24 hours a day shall exactly cover all proper items of expenditure, one does muddle one's whole life indefinitely. We never shall have any more time. We have, and we have always had, all the time there is.

CHAPTER FIVE

MAKING TIME FOR FITNESS
&

**"If we did all the things we were capable of doing,
we would literally astound ourselves."
~Thomas Edison**

DO YOU HAVE THE TIME?

There are 168 hours in a week – everyone on the planet has the same allotted time. What makes the difference is how each of us uses that time. Our quality of life is a direct result of what we are doing with the hours we have been given. Let's break it down. Sleep takes 7 to 8 hours a day for a total of 49 to 56 hours. Work takes 8 to 10 hours a day for a total of 40 to 50 hours. Meals, at approximately 2 hours a day, use up a total of 14 hours. The grand total is 103 to 120.

We have a lot of choices when it comes to the 48 to 65 hours we can use for other activities. Unfortunately, too many of us choose to use our time in one of the least productive ways possible: the average North American watches 5 hours of TV a day for a total of 35 hours a week!

When it comes to health, fitness, and vitality, it doesn't take a huge chunk of time to get results. All it takes is the consistent application of efforts in a forward direction. Can you spare half an hour to 45 minutes 3 times a week for exercise? Not too much to ask, considering we are given 168 hours. (That's barely one percent of our time in a week!)

Some say the best time to start fitness with your kids is when they are very young. The next best time is now! Get the message? If you are thinking about something, then it is time to TAKE ACTION! T-N-T. (That means today, not tomorrow!)

FAMILY PLANNING

Most people hear the phrase "family planning" and think about preparing for parenthood. But in our house, it means sitting down together and planning the upcoming week. First, we schedule work and other priority commitments. Then we make time for workouts. (We train with weights together three to four times per week.) One night of the week is reserved for our romance/date night, which we take turns orchestrating. (Anything goes!)

"The results have been magical."
~Uche and Kary

We started this weekly family planning after dreaming and brainstorming for a whole year about the kind of life we wanted to create. We wanted to write a book about the area of health, fitness, and personal growth but kept procrastinating. It was so frustrating: we knew we had to get started, but we seemed to find every reason to put it off. We were missing a powerful reason and a sense of urgency. The powerful reason finally came to us when we saw friends of ours who were living out their dream life on the coast. They seemed so content and happy. We asked: "Why not us?"

Now that we had the reason, it was time to create some urgency. We created this urgency by giving ourselves deadlines and by allotting weekly time for setting our goals. The results have been magical. Obviously, the book got finished, and we are now living our passion by sharing our knowledge of fitness with others. And there isn't any reason you can't enjoy similar benefits.

"Strong reasons make strong actions."
~Shakespeare

COMMON EXCUSES FOR POSTPONING FITNESS

I don't have enough time! It often takes a major life-threatening event before someone will make time for fitness. But wouldn't it be better for us to establish stronger reasons and a sense of urgency *before* a crisis develops? Here's a little secret: you don't find time – you make time! Remember, time is a non-renewable resource, so value it instead of spending it wastefully. Give your day more thought with respect to how you are setting time aside for your body and mind management.

I can't afford it. Your valuable time should be accounted for even though you are not a CEO. You are the president of "You, Inc." Time is the great equalizer! Rich man, poor man, beggar man, thief: we all have our allotted 24 hours per day, 7 days per week. What separates the "doers" from the "watchers" is the effective use of that time.

I don't have time to plan. If you don't have time to plan, then you better have time for the pain of regret! The discipline of planning your day weighs ounces; the regret for not taking the time to make fitness a major priority weighs tons! It is amazing how many good excuses you can manufacture when you are not moving toward the things you would like to do. The 10 minutes taken once a week to plan your fitness time is vital. Sunday night is a perfect time to prepare for the coming week!

"Something came up – maybe I'll start next week." Before you know it, weeks and then years have gone by. The consequences slowly sneak up on you. It's like a nagging toothache. The pain and anguish could have been avoided by early prevention. However, what is easy to do is also easy not to do. And it is the postponing of the early prevention and maintenance that will cause problems in the future.

"What about my friends? I need to spend time with them." Take some time to re-evaluate the people you flock with: are they nurturing and supportive of your dreams? Are they Energy Givers or Energy Drainers? (See the chapter, "Who Is in Your Flock?") Would you knowingly choose to spend the last day on the planet with people who bring you down?

"I have so much to do. I'll get started next week." Can you imagine United States Senator Hilary Clinton, singer Celine Dion, or Bill Gates of Microsoft saying that? Waiting for the perfect time is a no-win situation. Write down your intentions. Prioritize! Make a "to-do" list, and circle or underline those things that are "musts" for this week. Do not start with the other things on the list until you have completed the MUSTS! Waiting for the perfect time can be paralysing. You have the power to make any time the right time.

"I have no physical problems, and I'm not suffering right now. Why should I exercise?" Is life about getting by? Is life about staying two steps ahead of the creditors, using coffee as fuel, or searching through the medicine cabinet for the antacids? No, it's not! Why not live the health and relationship good life? How about living a life where people are asking you for exercise tips?

"What about the KIDS?" We have interviewed many parents who manage to exercise, spend time alone with each other, and spend quality time with their children. Here are some of their tips:

- Share duties with another family. Take turns looking after each other's children.
- Make the kids a part of a fitness night out. Include activities they would like and that you would like (e.g., family skating, swimming, or bike riding).
- Join a facility that caters to all ages and provides programming for your children while you participate in your own activity.
- Be a role model. Taking the time for your own health will set the standard for your children's future. Your children are watching your every move.
- Avoid using your children as an excuse for not having time to invest in your own health. Children pick up on these messages and take them to heart!
- See time with your children as an opportunity to try new activities or re-learn activities you enjoyed when you were their age.
- Use suppertime as a family discussion time. Share your dreams and goals with your children. Have them share theirs!

DID YOU KNOW?
The incidence of childhood obesity has increased 60% in the past 30 years. Only one third of all children who live less than a mile from school actually walk to school.

TIME AS AN INVESTMENT

We will always spend more time on things we value. This fact has a few repercussions. If your finances are not in great shape, it's probably because you haven't been giving them significant time. If your relationships aren't in great shape, it's most likely because you haven't been spending quality time with the important people in your life. If your body isn't in the greatest shape, it's most likely because you haven't spent much time taking care of it.

How much time is needed? Enough time. What does that mean? Enough to earn and invest so you and your family can live the life you deserve. Enough to show the people around you that you care. Enough to take care of the body you have been given.

By simply asking yourself before you start any activity: "Is this the best use of my time right now? Is this activity going to bring me increased levels of health? Will it bring me closer to my loved ones?" Good questions stimulate good answers. Time, a non-renewable resource, is one of our most valuable gifts.

MANAGING YOUR TIME

Many North Americans are working more and enjoying less free time. We have listed some easy ways for you to free up more time for yourself to do the things you want to do:

1. Check and respond to your e-mails once per day. Approximately 120 million people in North America have e-mail. Constantly checking on your e-mail is like having letters delivered to your home one at a time and opening them as they come in. You may feel like you're busy, but it is not the best use of your time.

2. Shorten your paper trail. We each get almost 3,000 pieces of mail a year. Our recommendation? Touch each piece of mail only once, and ask yourself if it ought to be thrown out or dealt with.

3. Go to bed! Two-thirds of us are not getting enough sleep. If you are overtired, you will lack the concentration to complete tasks promptly. Therefore, get a good seven to eight hours of sleep each night.

4. Work harder at work. It is amazing that only 60% of our 8-hour days are productive. Try increasing your pace instead of staying longer at the office or taking work home. Productivity plunges 25% when people work more than 60 hours per week.

5. Simplify your life. Downsize the number of things you have to look after. De-junk your home. Having less stuff means more time to enjoy what's really important—health and fitness and the special people in your life.

DEVELOPING TIME CONSCIOUSNESS

"I have seen who I can be. I must act to make it so."
~Greg Anderson, author of *Living Life on Purpose*

It is important to develop time consciousness. Using time wisely and setting time aside for health is an important statement to the Universe that you value yourself. Time mastery leads to life mastery! Consider the following tools to help you master your time and your life.

A Calendar. We keep a corkboard with 12 calendar pages posted in our home office, so we can view our major events, trips, and goals for the year. A year can fly by quickly. Why not make each day count? These calendar pages can be saved forever as documentation of your family's accomplishments!

A Day Planner. It's ironic that we will make very detailed plans for vacations, but not for our health and fitness. Having a written game plan would allow you to keep your vision alive.

A Journal. We wrote earlier about creating a journal where your dreams, goals, and memories can be chronicled.

A Project Book. Divide a binder or notebook into sections that represent the important areas of your life – physical, spiritual, financial, social, family, intellectual for example. If you have any new projects that will involve one of those areas, write them in the appropriate section. Whenever you take some action on those projects, make notes in that section. With the structure of a project book, you will be able to see more accurately how you are allocating your time to the different areas of your life.

> **"Well-arranged time is the truest marker of**
> **a well-arranged mind."**
> **~Sir Isaac Pitman**

Do you really need a journal, a day planner, a calendar, or a project book? No. You don't if all you want to do is just get by. Our challenge to you is to activate one or two of the time-management tools from this chapter immediately. You will discover that once they become a part of your daily ritual, you will enjoy many positive benefits. Remember, it could be the next thing you try that could make all the difference in the world.

JOURNAL ACTIVITY

Can you think of a few ways that you could manage time better, thus freeing up more time for health and fitness?

"Love cures people –
both the ones who give it
and the ones who receive it."
~Dr. Karl Menninger

CHAPTER SIX

WHO IS IN YOUR FLOCK?

ဢ

"We are each of us angels with only one wing,
and we can only fly embracing each other."
~Luciano de Crescenzo

"I've learned that meeting interesting people
depends less on where you go than who you are."
~H. Jackson, *Live and Learn and Pass It On*

THE POWER OF RELATIONSHIPS

The old saying "birds of a feather flock together" definitely has merit. The leading experts in human performance tell us if we want to enjoy more success, we'd better start spending time with successful people. Why? Because our relationships have tremendous influence on us.

"We live our lives as reflections of the
expectations of our peers."
~Anthony Robbins

If we spend the majority of our time with people who enjoy active lifestyles, it's easier to start incorporating healthy practices into our own lives. Did you know that psychological research has shown that we can only admire traits in others that we ourselves possess? In other words, if you admire a friend's disciplined pursuit of fitness, then you yourself have the potential to develop that same discipline also. If you didn't have this potential, you wouldn't even notice it.

It makes sense that this concept applies (perhaps even more) to couples. Doesn't it seem right to have someone in your life that you admire and respect? Out of this mutual admiration you will treat each other with greater care. We feel that one of life's greatest gifts is one person caring for another.

> **"Our friends see the best in us, and by that**
> **very fact, call forth the best from us."**
> **~Hugh Black**

The benefits of having this elevated type of relationship are many: feeling emotionally safe; being able to express your thoughts, dreams, and goals without judgment; and being able to encourage and support each other's personal evolution. We feel it's possible for anyone to have an exquisite bond and enjoy its ripple effect in every aspect of his or her life.

> **"When two spider webs unite,**
> **they can tie up a lion!"**
> **~African proverb**

SYNERGY

Once you harness the "power of two," there is no stopping what you can do! Stephen Covey's concept of synergy states that when two people come together in harmony, a more effective outcome will be achieved than either could have accomplished alone. 1 + 1 can add up to 2, but if you try looking at it with synergy in mind: 1 and 1 can become 11.

> *"We realized how much more we could*
> *achieve together than alone."*
> *~Kary*

Uche and I have always been people who strive for more in life. We both had full lives before we met - we were actively helping others in our professions, and we had many interesting and exciting plans for the future. As individuals, we were both pretty happy. Life was good!

When we met, it was like a lightning bolt had hit! Good turned into AMAZING! Both of us realized how much more we could achieve together. We were a united front working together toward our dreams and goals.

SUPPORT EACH OTHER'S FITNESS PURSUITS

> **"Love is not a competitive sport"**
> **~Leo Buscaglia**

1. Discuss your mental picture of health and fitness. Do not judge or argue whose version is more accurate. An important defining trait of any close and fulfilling relationship is finding and building common ground.

2. Assist each other in rediscovering an unrealized wish from childhood. You can then nurture and support a long-forgotten dream to dance or to run a marathon. Hey ladies – if you are looking to improve your fitness level and your husband or boyfriend is not interested, maybe the best thing to do is to find out what sport he liked when he was in high school. If it was hockey, then buy some skates and take him to the nearest rink! Hey guys – if your wife or girlfriend is not too interested in weight training and you would like to try something active together – then maybe it's time for the ballroom dancing lessons she's been hinting about for the past two years!

3. If you have a reluctant significant other, your desire to help may simply be put into action by setting a good example. Never give up on them! As you begin to notice your own positive benefits—share them with your spouse. If you see a glimmer of interest, then encourage it and ask them to join you.

**"We are not held back by the love we did not receive in the past,
but by the love we are not extending in the present."
~Marianne Williamson**

4. Give each other praise anytime you take a healthy step forward. By making deposits in your emotional bank accounts, you encourage each other to take further action. Long before toned muscles appear and excess pounds disappear, you can genuinely nurture and appreciate each other's efforts.

5. Be flexible in scheduling your shared fitness activities. We meet four days per week at the gym right after work. It may not be the "perfect time" for both of us, and we have to go in separate vehicles because we come from opposite ends of the city, but we are guaranteed four quality hours per week together! Flexibility in your scheduling is as important as working on the flexibility of your body.

**"Over the years I've learned that nobody makes it alone.
Every one of us gets through the tough times
because somebody is there, standing in the gap to close it for us."
~Oprah Winfrey**

POSITIVE ROLE MODELS

It is very important for children to see their parents taking care of themselves and enjoying life. Shakti Gawain, in her book *Living in the Light*, says that for many parents, having children is an easy excuse to neglect their own needs. Fitness is usually one of the first things to go when schedules are hectic.

But consider this: children are masters of observation. If they see their parents enjoying fitness activities, they are more likely to make it part of their everyday lives. Practicing sound nutrition and engaging in fun fitness activities with your children could add an entirely new dimension to your own enjoyment.

SOMETHING TO THINK ABOUT
Have you ever noticed that young people are pure potential? Whenever you have the opportunity, fill them with "possibility thinking" and encourage them to set lofty goals. A powerful practice is to role model positive behaviours without lecturing.

---

*"Family can create a powerful reason to become
more than you already are."*
~Uche

When I hear the word flock, I think of closeness, protection, and a fully functioning unit. I think back to times when I felt very connected to my family, and my world seemed simple and predictable. I remember some specific times when our family would have special discussions after dinner. My two brothers, one sister and I would be finished eating, and we would be anxious to run outside and play. My father and mother would have us stay at the table and talk in turn about our day. We would each get a turn (awkwardly at first) to give the family a rundown of what happened in school.

Over time, it got easier. We had no problem describing what we did, where we went, and what we had learned. Many times we would tease each other and receive a stern look from our father. It was that look that let us know in no uncertain terms that he took this exercise very seriously. It made us feel good to know he was listening and that what we said had value.

I remember trying not to look too interested while I listened to my sister talk. But I found myself being drawn into the drama of her day and being totally enraptured by her message. I found myself leaning forward as she described her activities. She had a unique way of looking at life and I really did love her stories.

It was those special times that drew our family even closer together. It was that early connection that gave me a strong, solid core belief in the power of family.

ENERGY GIVERS

Energy Givers are those people in our lives who challenge us to raise our sights even higher. They focus on our strengths (which we sometimes do not see) and give unconditional support and love, even when we're engulfed by the darkness of "self-doubt."

There are many benefits to spending time with the Energy Givers in our lives. Their enthusiasm for their own projects and interests is contagious.

"Alone we can do so little;
together we can do so much."
~Helen Keller

We saw this firsthand when freelance writer, Martin Zeilig, interviewed us for a local newspaper story on couples and fitness. We admired the man's work, his expertise with words, and his enthusiasm. A mutual admiration and friendship developed. We would meet to discuss our current projects and found that we could all help each other with our plans and dreams. There is nothing more amazing than being able to share ideas with someone who will support and nurture your thoughts.

"There are two parts to influence:
First, influence is powerful; and second, influence is subtle.
You wouldn't let someone push you off course, but you might let
someone nudge you off course and not even realize it."
~Jim Rohn

ENERGY DRAINERS

Do you have friends or family members who never have anything positive to say? Have you noticed that they zap your energy and leave you feeling drained and uncomfortable? Your inner voice warns you every time, but you still hope the next meeting will be better than the last.

"Do not be deceived, bad company corrupts good morals."
~1 Corinthians 15:33 (NASB)

Do you have people in your life who seem to have a knack for letting everyone around them know what *isn't* possible? Remember that the people who tell you it cannot be done are often the people who cannot see it happening in their own lives. They are simply projecting their own inabilities or feelings of inadequacy onto you.

Inspirational speaker and corporate trainer Les Brown has a great response to these folks: **"What you think about me is none of my business."**

It would be fantastic to be able to replay these words in our minds whenever we are on the receiving end of another's negative broadcast. Everyone is entitled to his or her opinion. But, the key word here is *opinion*. It only becomes a fact if we buy into it.

"All communication comes from a place of love or is a cry for help."
~Marianne Williamson

Of course, everyone deserves a second chance, but when do you draw the line? Energy Drainers constantly complain about their lives but never take any action. In addition, they may constantly remind you of your failures, possibly thwarting your attempts to move ahead. They may even try to convince you that you should be satisfied with the way things are.

Negative comments, gossip, hateful words, lies, judgments, and putdowns are all cries for help. They are projections of emotional pain and inner turmoil. It is easy to react negatively when someone attacks your efforts. In the moment, remember that the person is speaking from their own limited view and may not be able to show encouragement for something they don't believe is possible for themselves.

This strategy takes a lot of practice! It is human nature to react when you feel threatened. It is easy to fall back to immobilizing patterns when someone negates your efforts. Can you recall a time when you were so angered by someone's comments that you were reduced to tears or felt like giving up on your dream? Can you now see a new way to look at the situation?

"Get around people who have something of value to share with you. Their impact will continue to have a significant effect on your life long after they have departed."
~Jim Rohn

WHERE DO YOU STAND?

Have you ever considered which category you typically fit in? Are you a Drainer or a Giver? Congratulations if you spend most of your time being a Giver! One of the true joys in life is the knowledge that you have added value to the lives of others.

If you realize you are a Drainer, don't be discouraged. Simple awareness can begin the process of change. Consider the following ten characteristics of Energy Givers:

1. They are passionately involved in activities and careers they love.
2. Their passion is contagious and motivating.
3. They have an unconscious competence about their actions—they make things look easy.
4. They live their lives without seeking approval.
5. Their faces glow with an unmistakable light: they stand out in a crowd.
6. They look for the positive qualities in others, and they find it easy to give compliments.
7. They give you their full attention when you are with them.
8. They are committed to their own self-improvement and the improvement of society.
9. They usually have interesting stories and insights into the human condition.
10. They are open-minded.

> **"Friendship is a word the very sight
> of which in print makes the heart warm."**
> **~Augustine Birrell**

How does a person become an Energy Giver in the world of fitness? There are many ways. You can begin by taking care of yourself. By following sound nutritional practices, getting sufficient rest, and staying active, you are in a better position to positively influence others in your sphere. Become known for encouraging and supporting others' efforts to get fit. Likewise, it is vital to have unconditional love and compassion for those in your inner circle who are doing their best with what they have been given. We are all on our own paths in this life: we have different talents and abilities, and it is not fair to expect everyone to be as motivated as you at all times.

A new commitment to health and fitness is fragile in its beginning stages. It is very easy to get off track. Did you know that it takes 21 to 30 days for a new behaviour to become a habit? In the early stages, it is very important to strengthen your own resolve and nurture your new healthy choices daily. This may mean only sharing with Energy Givers – not everyone around you!

> **"There is only one corner of the
> universe you can be certain of improving,
> and that is your own self."**
> **~Aldous Huxley**

HEALTHY NUTRITION FOR OUR MINDS

If you do not have any Energy Givers or positive role models in your life, then read about them! An uplifting biography can be a great way to tune into the mindset of people who have reached the summit. Let your imagination work wonders while you read! With every autobiography and biography, we are given an intimate look into a person's life we may never get a chance to meet. Miracles await all those who can make reading an integral part of their lives. Books played key roles in the success stories of

Oprah Winfrey, Sylvester Stallone, Arnold Schwarzenegger, Maya Angelou, and Anthony Robbins, to name only a few.

SIX WAYS TO IMPROVE YOUR FLOCK

"To show a child what has once delighted you, to find the child's delight added to your own, so that there is now a double delight seen in the glow of trust and affection: this is happiness."
~J.B. Priestley

- Expose your *current flock* to new things like eating sushi or entering a family fun run.

- Circulate with new groups that are stimulating and uplifting—try toastmasters or join a running club.

- Contribution is a great way to enhance our human experience. Donate blood, sponsor a foster child, or volunteer at the Special Olympics. You'll meet many interesting and inspiring people.

- Select friends who stand above petty, unimportant things.

- Ask successful people for advice. They usually enjoy sharing their experiences.

- Ask yourself the question, "Where are my current friends leading me?" It is important to have relationships with people who inspire, uplift, or bring out the best in you. Don't think for a moment that you can spend time with people and not be affected or influenced by their beliefs.

"Whoever walks with the wise grows wise;
whoever mixes with fools will be ruined."
~Proverbs 13:20

JOURNAL ACTIVITY

Who are the people in your life who are Energy Givers? When was the last time you told them how much their influence means to you?

Who do you have a direct influence on? How could you become a better role model for these people?

> **"The greatest happiness of life is the conviction**
> **that we are loved."**
> **~Victor Hugo**

SUGGESTED READING:

The Path to Love, by Deepak Chopra
Spiritual insights are applied to relationships. He beautifully illustrates how our lives can be transformed by bringing spirit into love.

CHAPTER SEVEN

FOOD FOR FUNCTION- STRAIGHT TALK
ಬಂ

**"Take care of your stomach the first 50 years, and it will take
care of you the last 50 years."
~Dr. Steven Smith**

Most people feel there's some special secret to healthy eating or living with the principles of sound nutrition. What is the secret to healthy eating? Well, the secret is: there is no secret! Sorry to disappoint you.

It is our goal to demystify the subject and show you that eating with healthy principles requires a little self-discipline, an open mind, and most importantly, enjoying the process. Seeing food for what it really is – fuel for energy and growth – is one of the most important parts of gaining mastery.

The topic of eating is a hot one no matter how you slice it. The main purpose of food is to fuel the body. But for many people, the relationship with food goes far beyond pure function. Family gatherings and celebrations are seen as a time to indulge. Time with friends is often spent over lunch or dinner. Romantic evenings are often long, drawn out gustatory affairs. Even in the workplace, we're bombarded with treats in the staff room – does it not seem like some good soul is bringing baked goods or birthday cake at least once a week?

It seems like we are in a never-ending cycle of planning meals, preparing meals, serving meals, cleaning up after meals, or shopping for next week's meals. Throw in the discussions about where to go for dinner, and your life may seem like it revolves around food!

If only it were as easy to exercise as it is to eat!

*"Christmas is a time of year when life
revolves around food in our family."*
~Kary

There is a continual flurry of food preparation and feasting during the holidays. Whenever I think back to past Christmas celebrations, my thoughts are smothered with decadent homemade fudge and shortbread cookies. I can remember the exact layout of the dessert table, which was always laden with the most exquisite, mouth-watering treats.

I have made many changes in my lifestyle over the past years— now fitness and good nutrition are very important to me. I exercise regularly and make a conscious effort to choose nutritious foods. Yet amazingly, every year during the Christmas season, I fall victim to thoughts of gorging on sweets. I guess old habits die hard!

Fit for the Love of It! was written with the intention of helping you uncover powerful reasons to make permanent lifestyle changes. There's always new information and findings to consider. Don't worry: we're not going to burden you with complex formulas and technical terms. You probably know enough already to start living a healthy existence. The challenge is that people don't act on what they know.

Is there a gap between where you are health-wise and where you want to be? Our goal is to help you bridge that gap. We are able to help because we've been there – just starting out, unsure, and maybe a little overwhelmed. In order to make "the leap of faith", you must have powerful reasons to get to the other side.

**Treat your body like a temple- a place you honour and respect. It's not
an outhouse! Learn how to care for it,
and it will serve you well now and into the future.**

INFORMATION OVERLOAD

Never before in the history of humankind have we had such a large quantity of information about the human body. Only in the last 30 years has there been intense research and a better understanding of the effects of nutrition on our health, aging, and athletic performance. There are tens of thousands of articles, research papers, and books available on the subject. We're faced not with a lack of information but with an overwhelming amount of it!

> **"Information overload leads to burnout,**
> **which leads to tuning out,**
> **which can end up in a pig out!"**
> **~Carolyn O'Neil (former CNN health correspondent)**

OVEREATING

> *"Impulsive eating set me up for plenty of problems."*
> *~Cary C.*

We've all been told at some point by a family doctor or well-meaning relative that we should be eating to live, rather than living to eat. I'll be the first to admit I love food. In essence, I live to eat. Sadly, that means food is equated with immediate pleasure for me, not function. It starts off with a simple mouth-watering signal to the brain after a TV commercial or a billboard I pass on the way to work featuring a larger-than-life cheeseburger I just have to try. Or the urge to splurge may just simply fill an emotional need—from loneliness to depression. Whatever the case, I've got to get to the nearest drive thru and satiate my desire.

There's no concern over consequences. Immediate gratification is the only goal. This becomes an extremely dangerous cycle. Compounded over time, the damage is irreversible. Impulsive eating sets me up for plenty of problems . . .

Overeating is a condition that has existed since the beginning of time. If you look back some 100,000 years (long before the drive-thru restaurant), there was no government to regulate production and storage of food. Refrigeration did not exist, so in times of excess, people engaged in frenzied eating to celebrate. And in times of famine, the extra bodyfat was an asset.

There are health consequences to overeating. Your entire digestive system must work overtime. It takes a massive amount of energy to break down a large volume of food into its useable components. Your body won't have as much energy for activities such as communicating, problem solving, or standing upright.

Are you constantly tired or wonder why you don't have the energy you ought to? Do you rely on coffee or other caffeinated drinks to get through the day? Is your concentration lacking at certain times of the day? Do you experience heartburn, indigestion, bloating, fatigue, mood swings, or flatulence? Or, have long-term consequences become your daily battle: obesity, diabetes, heart disease, loss of mobility, joint problems, poor self-image, eating disorders, social isolation, depression, or even cancer?

Most people are aware of these risk factors, yet they regularly overeat. They try justifying their behaviour by saying: "I missed breakfast," "It's a special occasion," "It's free," "My eyes were bigger than my stomach," or "I can't let it go to waste; there are people starving in some parts the world."

Obviously this is an area that needs to be addressed! Unless the underlying reasons are identified, you may always find yourself unbuckling your belt at the dinner table.

"I have to admit I am in love with food.
I eat until I get tired, and then I drift off to sleep.
I sleep until I'm hungry enough to wake up.
I've got a nice rhythm going."
~Comedian Glen Foster

EMOTIONAL EATING AND CRAVINGS

We eat when we're hungry. But, we also tend to eat when we're stressed, bored, unhappy, anxious, or lonely. Perhaps we eat to temporarily take our minds off our woes. With a pail of ice cream and soup spoon in hand, we can completely get immersed in the physical moment. Breathing deepens, colours brighten, and a feeling of euphoria fills us. Memories of happier times and feelings often flood back. Feel-good hormones saturate our brains. And we link all these feelings to the *food*.

It doesn't take a degree in psychology to see that food helps us cope. Who hasn't gone to the fridge for some ice cream when they're down in the dumps? It very easily becomes a habit to head for the kitchen whenever we feel things are not going well. And why does it seem like the foods we crave are always the ones that are high in sugar? How often have you reached for a head of lettuce when you're feeling blue? Elizabeth Somer, R.D., wrote about this connection in *Food & Mood*. She emphasized that it's only a temporary fix, and if done often enough, it can lead to unwanted weight gain.

Cravings are not a true indicator of hunger. Taking the time to ask yourself what you're really feeling can help you deal with the problem. Ask yourself if you're hungry or just bored.

No volume of food will curb the craving if the root cause is not dealt with. Dr. Deepak Chopra, author of *Ageless Body, Timeless Mind*, says that simple awareness of the personal challenge at hand can initiate healing. There's no shame in receiving counselling if that's what it takes to break out of the prison of destructive feelings and behaviours. Author and speaker Les Brown says, "What you resist will persist." In other words, you may end up thinking about the *demon doughnuts* all day if you never address the real issue.

JOURNAL ACTIVITY

Describe the effects your present eating habits have on your life and your health.

Who else in your life is affected by your food choices?

What kind of health challenges could you possibly have in the future if you don't make any changes?

How does that make you feel?

Close your eyes for a minute and breathe deeply.
Let these feelings sink in.

Is this the kind of legacy you want to leave behind?

Are you ready to make some new decisions about your relationship with food?

TRY LIFESTYLE EATING INSTEAD OF DIETING

> **"God doesn't require us to be successful;**
> **he only requires that we try."**
> **~Mother Teresa**

Just mentioning the word "diet" sends shivers down people's spines. It reeks of restriction and suffering. Look at the word itself: diet or **DIE**-IT has morbid overtones.

There's nothing mysterious or magical about decreasing your bodyweight on any diet. One thing they have in common is the restriction of calories. Let us ask you: can any one diet promise permanent weight loss? No. You will keep the weight off only as long as you're on that particular diet. The moment you leave the restrictions of the diet, the weight creeps (or somersaults) back on. But if you change your habits – your lifestyle – you *can* make a permanent change.

Lifestyle eating is the term we like to use. It refers to sound nutrition as a way of life rather than some short-term dietary eating plan.

"Never eat anything at one sitting that you can't lift."
~Miss Piggy

COMBATTING YOUR CRAVINGS

1. Don't skip meals. Skipping meals leads to over-eating at the first available opportunity. It also leads to making unhealthy choices.

2. At most meals, aim to eat carbohydrates (like brown rice, whole-grain products, and vegetables) with protein (for example, chicken, fish, lean red meat, eggs). This will help you enjoy sustained energy and feel more satisfied.

3. Try deep breathing and relaxation techniques if and when any cravings start.

4. Exercise. You could go for a walk or a jog to get your legs moving and heart pumping. Movement will also raise levels of your body's own feel-good chemicals (endorphins). Not only does exercise feel good, it's hard to wolf down potato chips when you're on the treadmill.

5. Listen to music. It can change the way you feel – energize you if you're bored or relax you if you're stressed.

6. Phone someone. A good conversation with a friend can help distract you from any craving – unless they're working at a take-out restaurant.

7. A pact or fun contract with your significant other could inspire you to new disciplinary heights.

8. Drink plenty of water. You would be surprised how often people mistake dehydration for hunger!

Bill Phillips, best-selling author of Body-*for*-LIFE, suggests having a "free day" or a "cheat day" once a week. On this day, you allow yourself to eat anything you desire. He reports that there's a physiological benefit to doing this. This strategy convinces our bodies that we're not starving. Plus, it gives us a psychological boost – imparting a sense of freedom from any perceived restriction.

> **"You have an innate desire to eat,**
> **but you don't have an innate desire for a particular food."**
> ~Yefim Shubentsov, author of *Cure Your Cravings*

JUST SAY NO!

Develop your mental gymnastics. If a torte or a honey-glazed doughnut tempts you, remember your decision to choose healthier food. Ask yourself if a poor choice will work against your new health and fitness goals. Just saying "NO" strengthens self-discipline. It feels good to walk away from a dessert or a high-calorie treat. You can walk a little taller knowing you're better than the doughnut. Okay, we're getting a little silly. But the point is to say "NO" to debauchery and "YES" to sound nutrition.

CONSIDER THIS:
We love the story about the prize racehorse who gets exactly the right amount of calories, vitamins, minerals, exercise, and rest he needs for his optimal champion performance. The owner has spent plenty of money and time purchasing, feeding, and caring for this animal.
The owner? Well, he just came through a drive-thru, smoked two cigarettes, and is looking forward to the banquet on the night of the horse's victory. How many of us take better care of our animals than we do ourselves?

BE PATIENT

Eating healthy and maintaining an exercise program all year round does get easier as time goes on. You don't have to give up your friends, families, and social functions but, it takes time to get comfortable with new eating strategies: you have spent many years adapting your body to your current eating habits, so don't expect to make too many changes overnight.

You'll begin to see and feel results in time. It's human nature to want it all NOW. This is the time to reflect back to the powerful reasons that inspired you to make those new decisions. Hopefully these reasons are more powerful than the numbers on the scale. If they aren't, you'll need to re-evaluate why the results have become more important than the reasons.

> **"First say to yourself what you would be;**
> **and then do what you have to do."**
> **~Epictetus, Greek philospher**

We know you are excited, but trying to add too many new behaviours at one time can be overwhelming, which makes the entire process tedious. The biggest consequence of setting impossible standards is disappointment, which most often leads to giving up altogether. Gradual changes made with a conscious effort can last a lifetime.

> *"During the second week, I began wondering*
> *when the miraculous transformation would take place.*
> *How come I still looked the same?"*
> *~Andrew*

I was sick and tired of the way I looked and felt. I tried to do everything at once. I gave up my coffee, I threw out my cookies, and I vowed to never eat chocolate again! Bye-bye banana splits. I hired a trainer and saw a registered dietician. I purchased a membership at my local gym and a treadmill for my 6:00 am cardio workout.

For the first week, I managed to exercise two hours per day and did not veer from my established eating plan. During the second week, I began wondering when the miraculous transformation would take place. How come I still looked the same?

My family was feeling alienated by my Navy Seals training regimen—even the dog was avoiding me. By the end of the second week, I found myself in a drive-thru wolfing down a double burger, fries, and a shake.

FIGHT STRESS WITH HEALTHY NUTRITION

Stress is a common ailment in our fast-paced world. Our primitive ancestors used the stress response – fight or flight – for survival. But in modern times, this primitive response is activated daily from less than deadly situations (e.g., getting caught in a traffic jam, waiting to de-board a plane, someone cutting in front of you in the buffet line … the list is infinite). In primitive times, fighting or fleeing relieved the stress. This doesn't work too well at the airport ticket counter!

Without regular activity, stress will linger in your system and take its toll on your body. Stress can deplete certain nutrients—Vitamin C, iron, and calcium, for example. If you experience a lot of stress in your life, nutritious food choices are a must.

FEED YOUR MIND WITH EMPOWERING INFORMATION

Find tasty recipes for good health, and concentrate on becoming your own nutrition guru. There are hundreds of books available. Acquiring knowledge in an area that's important to you is intoxicating. Each book you read will only increase your passion for learning. Keep an open mind, and do not stop at one source. You can learn at least one thing from each book, even if you don't agree with everything in it.

Don't overlook the internet for increasing your storehouse of knowledge. There's an abundance of great nutrition websites. Use the following guidelines as you browse to weed out inappropriate information:

- Do the claims sound too good to be true?
- Is there a promise of a quick fix?
- Are certain food groups omitted?
- Are there severe or unrealistic restrictions?
- Are references included for any health claims?

STRIVE FOR EXCELLENCE, NOT PERFECTION

Give up that all-or-nothing attitude! We often hear people say that once they have eaten one cookie, they may as well finish the entire row. This all-or-nothing mindset often leads to a whole day of bingeing. Having one cookie does not mean you have "blown" your decision to eat healthy! Do not write off a day because you overate at one meal! Re-affirm your healthy intentions, and move forward. **Remember – strive for excellence, not perfection!**

EAT INTUITIVELY

A study in the New England Journal of Medicine found that pre-school children could intuitively regulate how much they ate according to their bodies' requirements for growth. As adults, can we follow the lead of our children and eat more intuitively?

At mealtime, ask yourself if the food you are about to eat will be helping or hindering you in your quest for better health. Another recommendation is to eat well 90% of the time with Food for Function in mind. This will allow for those special occasions and times when it is almost impossible to say no (like on your birthday!).

"All personal breakthroughs begin with a change in beliefs."
~Anthony Robbins

EAT MINDFULLY

Eat slowly in a relaxed atmosphere. It takes about 20 minutes for the stomach to signal the brain that it's full. Eating quickly will often lead to overeating, so try to put your fork down between bites. Make an effort to chew slowly and enjoy the taste of your food. You will get more satisfaction and better nutritional value if you take the time to chew your food properly. Jonathan Goldman (author of *Healing Sounds*) suggests listening to slow music while you dine.

DID YOU KNOW?
48% of North Americans are overweight or obese

Avoid other activities while eating. Watching television will only distract you from your meal and tempt you with mouth-watering commercials. Try to eat at the table instead of standing at the counter reading the mail and returning your phone calls.

"To this day, I have to remind myself to slow down..."
~Uche

Because I come from a large family, this recommendation is still a tough one for me. Growing up with two brothers and a sister, it was a race to see who would finish first, so they could get seconds. To this day, I have to remind myself to slow down.

NIX THE QUICK FIX

Avoid quick fixes or fad diets. Any plan that limits or restricts certain food groups or calories will only be effective while you are on it. Did you know that 95% of dieters regain lost weight within two years?

"I'm heavier now than when I first started riding the diet roller-coaster."
~Jill

I'm a walking nutritional database. I have tried every diet on the market. I can tell you about fat grams, calories, glycemic index... you name it. I'm heavier now than when I first started riding the diet roller-coaster. And I'm preoccupied with the enemy – food.
I go out for dinner with friends or family and put up a brave front. I pick at a plain, lifeless salad and eat very little. Later on, I eat alone in the comfort of my home, where I can eat whatever I want. I feel stuck. I cannot bear the thought of going on another diet, but I still want to lose weight.

Obsessively controlling food adds a false sense of structure and certainty to a day. Chronic dieters get the opportunity to feel special every time they explain their new regimens. When the quick fix ends with failure, the dieter often receives consolation and connection with others who have also "fallen off the wagon." This becomes a seductive, but vicious cycle.

DON'T SKIP MEALS

When you skip meals, you deny yourself the regular intake of fuel and nutrients you require to function efficiently. Meal skippers tend to experience many energy highs and lows in their days. They may actually feel light-headed or irritable after not eating for many hours.

Have you ever skipped breakfast because you're too rushed? Have you ever missed lunch while working toward a deadline? Have you missed meals because of an irregular schedule (e.g., shift work, holidays)? Have you ever missed meals because of stress? It's often an unconscious act, but it does have consequences.

Research has shown meal skippers are more likely to be overweight because they overeat later in the day to compensate for the missed meals. Meal skippers often have poor eating habits, which, combined with stress, can leave them vulnerable to illness. Skipping breakfast can lead to unhealthy choices later in the morning that often contain high amounts of sugar or caffeine.

START THE DAY OFF RIGHT

Eating a healthy breakfast bumps up your metabolism in the morning and helps complete the digestive process from the day before. For people not used to it, this can be a challenging habit to develop, but the payoff is worth it. You can start with just a piece of fruit or one of those new delicious meal-replacement shakes.

Are you still thinking, "Who needs breakfast? I get my early morning kick from coffee." Did you know that coffee gives you a false energy boost and can be addictive and dehydrating? Seventy percent of soft drinks also contain caffeine. Beware! Being a caffeine junkie can lead to headaches, anxiety, and insomnia. So, avoid using coffee to replace a meal, and enjoy it in moderation. (May we suggest one or two cups with a loved one in front of the fire?)

Did you know your body requires more fuel during the first half of the day than it does as it winds down for the evening? "Eat breakfast like a king; eat lunch like a lord; and supper like a pauper." What happens when you do the reverse? Well, people who tend to eat more during the second half of the day are more prone to storing the food as bodyfat. Brad King, author of *Fat Wars*, reported that optimal fat-burning can occur if you go to bed on an empty stomach. This best-selling author goes onto say that this habit will lead to excellent health, growth, repair, and slow the aging process.

EAT YOUR FRUITS AND VEGGIES

Fruits and vegetables are some of the richest nutrient powerhouses of the food groups. Including them in your daily intake is one of the keys to a treasure chest of vitality. Plant food provides a rich source of antioxidants and phytochemicals—substances that possess many health-protective benefits. An increase in the amount of these substances in the diet has been linked with the prevention and/or treatment of heart disease, cancer, diabetes, and a host of other medical conditions.

Research has shown that people who consume five to ten servings of fruit and vegetables have *half the risk* of developing cancer (e.g., you could achieve 5 servings by choosing: half a banana, a small apple, a half cup baby carrots, a small salad, and a half cup steamed broccoli). And, if they do get cancer, their chances of dying are decreased. Fruits and vegetables are also naturally low in cholesterol, saturated fats, and sodium, which have all been linked to heart disease.

Cancer and heart disease are the top two killers in North America, and they come with a hefty price tag. The mental and emotional strain of intense treatment weighs heavily on a family. The financial cost to the medical system is astronomical – over $45,000 for a heart bypass!

Eating fruits and vegetables is the most inexpensive and proactive way to prevent these conditions. Purchasing and preparing them is a daily affirmation of the importance of the health of your family. A bag of ready-cut spinach is only $2.00! An apple will set you back less than 30 cents!

Another tip is to eat your vegetables first. These low-calorie, nutrient-dense foods will fill you up. After you eat these, you will be satisfied with less of the higher calorie items on the table. Don't you think that this is a better alternative to having your stomach surgically stapled to stop you from overeating?

DID YOU KNOW?

The stomach is a very flexible organ. Overeating stretches the stomach beyond its natural size. It will not return to its natural size if it is constantly (at every meal) being stretched beyond its limits. This larger stomach will require more and more food to satisfy your perceived hunger. When you begin to eat with sound nutritional principles, it will take a while before that stretched stomach starts to regain its natural dimensions. That is why the first few weeks of nutritious eating may seem very challenging. We guarantee that over time, your body will get used to the new amounts of food – you will feel satisfied with smaller portions.

FIND OUT WHAT'S INSIDE

Checking food labels is a great habit. Taking the time to read them means you're taking responsibility for what goes into your body. By examining the labels, you will see the chemical additives, salt, sugar, and fat content of what you're eating. By simply being aware of the ingredients in your food, you'll make better choices. You'll begin to ask yourself the question, "Will this food item take me closer to the way I want to look and feel or further away?" This question can make the entire shopping experience much easier and more interesting.

> **"Never buy an item that has ingredients you can't pronounce or that say, 'Continued on the next can!'"**
> **~Marilu Henner, from her *Total Health Makeover***

CONTROL YOUR SERVING SIZE

We were eating at a nice Italian restaurant in Vancouver and couldn't help but overhear the conversation of the people at the next table. They didn't speak much during the entire dinner, other than to ask for more bread. The man groaned as he leaned back in his chair and placed his hands on his belly, obviously in great discomfort. His wife commiserated as she moaned: "Our eyes are always bigger than our stomachs!" He agreed and commented that everything looked so good he just didn't know when to stop.

Many of us are confused about how much food we should eat at each meal. The U.S.D.A. Food Pyramid and the Canada Food Guide recommend specific portion and serving sizes. For example, a serving of vegetables is the amount you could fit in half a regular coffee cup. (A salad would be a full cup.) A serving of meat would be the size of a deck of cards, and one serving of starchy carbohydrates (rice or pasta) would be half of a coffee cup. Beware: in this age of "SUPER-SIZE IT", it's possible to eat all your daily-recommended calories at one sitting!

If you are a grazer who continually goes into the kitchen and snacks in the evening until you go to bed, try recording everything you "snack" on for a few nights (include the quantity). Once you have this list, try placing everything you would eat in one evening on a table. You will then realize the quantity and quality of the food you're eating. You might need this wake-up call to see just how much you are eating every evening.

If you regularly overeat at one meal, your first step might be to limit yourself to only one serving (some of your plates might be stacked pretty high, but that's OK). After a few weeks, you will get used to your new habit of having only one serving. Remember to eat slowly, so you can stop eating before you are bursting at the seams. Your second step will be to load up your plate and make a conscious effort to remove a small portion before you begin eating. Perseverance will pay off, and you will eventually find that you require less food to fill up.

DECREASE YOUR UNHEALTHY FAT INTAKE

Reduce fat intake by taking note of the sources of food you're eating and consciously staying away from the higher fat content food sources. This can be accomplished by choosing leaner cuts of red meat, choosing your dairy products wisely, and selecting baked or grilled over fried foods. Using low-fat cooking sprays and non-stick pans in your food preparation will also help you on the road to living the good life.

Baked goods are often very high in unhealthy processed fats and should be limited. Brad King, in *Fat Wars,* calls these the "Frankenstein Fats." (Remember what Frankenstein looked like and how unhappy he was?) Studies showed that these fats are artificially altered to increase their shelf life and are more easily integrated into the cells of your body. It's reported they cause chaos and confusion in your cells. Recall the saying, "You are what you eat"?

It is simplistic to label all fats as bad. There are certain fats called essential fats (omega-3's and omega-6's) that are needed by the body for cell repair and the function of many organs. Your body will not perform well without these necessary fats. They have a direct impact: keeping your skin looking young, maintaining healthy hair, and promoting keen mental concentration. And for athletes, they are necessary for optimal performance. These "good" fats are the unsaturated fats, which are found in fish, nuts, flaxseed oil, and hemp oil, to name just a few.

HYDRATE FOR HEALTH

There are people in North America who may think they're ill, but actually, they're just thirsty. Science has demonstrated that increasing our water intake has positive effects on our energy levels, can help us shed excess pounds, and may help fight certain types of cancers. Water is one of the true magical elixirs of life.

About eight glasses a day is recommended. This may seem like a challenge in the beginning with the increase in bathroom breaks. However, after a few weeks of feeling and looking better with fresher breath, healthier skin, brighter eyes, better digestion, and increased energy, you will be convinced.

> **"Thousands have lived without love,**
> **not one without water."**
> ~W.H. Auden

GO LIGHT AT NIGHT

Stop eating about two to three hours before you go to bed. This gives your body a chance to digest most of the food before you go to sleep. If the body is trying to digest food while you're sleeping, your quality of rest will be reduced. So go to bed with your significant other, not a croissant!

DE-JUNK YOUR KITCHEN

Eliminate any food in your house that has not been chosen with sound nutritional principles. Now you'll avoid the midnight rendezvous with your refrigerator. You may be thinking: "What about the kids," or "We need to have treats for our guests." But consider this: if the average person ate three less cookies each day at 60 calories each with no other nutrition or exercise changes, he would lose around 10 pounds in a year!

Eating high-sugar treats can be very addictive. They are comfort foods. Sugar has been found to trigger the release of opiates (feel-good chemicals) in the brain. This high is short-lived and is followed by a crash in energy.

So get rid of the unhealthy treats that most households keep stockpiled. Who hasn't finished an entire bag of potato chips during a TV movie and then exclaimed: "I can't believe I ate all of that?" Having no junk in your house might sound extreme, but the results are amazing! The best part is you'll no longer have to feel uncomfortable when you eat that dessert at the restaurant or party if you have eaten with sound nutrition principles in mind all week!

"A shift in your personal mind-set is the key to all change.
We have to work on our inner dialogue and our personal habit
patterns before we implement changes in our lifestyles."
~Dee Hakala (winner of the Nike Fitness Innovation Award),
from her book *Thin is Just a Four Letter Word*

CHALLENGE:

Put down this book right now and take an inventory of your kitchen. Take everything that is considered "junk," and put it into a box and get rid of it. This will definitely be a challenge if you have been raised in a family with constant reminders of... "All the starving people in the world..."

If throwing it out bothers you, make some healthy donations to your local food bank! Foods laden with fat or sugar do not benefit anyone!

KEEP TRACK TO GET ON TRACK

In the beginning, it's worth it to keep a daily food journal. Record when and what you eat and how you were feeling before and after the food. A journal may help you eat more nutritious foods and identify underlying emotions you have with food. This could also be a great tool to identify vitamin and mineral deficiencies. You may be surprised at the reality of your daily eating habits—most people underestimate how many empty calories they eat and overestimate how many nutrient-rich foods are in their diets.

THE FURIOUS FOUR

Be aware of the furious four cell destroyers:

1. Sugar: Reduce or eliminate refined sugar in your diet. Too much sugar may lead to obesity, diabetes, and roller-coaster energy levels.

2. Tobacco: It's impossible to say you're healthy if you're a smoker. Benefits to quitting occur immediately. Did you know that after 24 hours, the risk for a heart attack decreases; after 2 to 3 weeks, lung function rises up to 30%; and after 1 to 9 months, coughing and fatigue decreases?

3. <u>Alcohol in excess</u>: It's toxic to the body and has many well-known side effects. In case you have forgotten some of them: it increases the chance of liver cancer, it ages you, and it destroys brain cells. (Whenever we misplace our vehicle in a large parking lot, we realize how few we have to spare!)

4. <u>Salt</u>: Reduce or eliminate the amount of table salt you use. Most people are taking in more than they need through food alone. Too much salt increases water retention and the chance of high blood pressure.

RESTAURANT SURVIVAL

Dining out at restaurants is an unavoidable part of today's world. John Naisbitt, in his bestseller *Megatrends 2000*, reported that 40 cents of every food dollar is spent in restaurants. We have compiled a list of suggestions that will help you face your next restaurant dining experience with anticipation rather than apprehension!

1. Before you leave for the restaurant, commit yourself to making healthier food choices. Pre-program yourself to eat with good nutritional principles before you set foot in the restaurant.

2. Do not go to a restaurant starving! It is a mistake to believe that skipping meals throughout the day gives you an excuse for overeating when you go out.

3. Enjoy your company more than the food! Think of dining out as a vehicle to get closer to the people you're with. Focussing on the conversation and your dining companions will enable you to eat slower.

4. Don't read the menu like you would a love letter. Menus are designed to tantalize and entice you into overeating.

5. Order with conviction. You set yourself up for failure the minute you waiver in your intention and start asking what other people are going to order. People admire someone who can make a quick decision. Certainty is very attractive! Take the lead and set the tone for a healthy meal. If you have children with you, remember they learn by watching. A lifetime of good eating habits begins at family mealtime. When dining out, they will follow your lead.

6. Ask for dressings and sauces (which contain many artery-clogging saturated fat calories) on the side, so you have control over the quantity you consume.

7. If your meal comes with bread, ask your server not to bring it. Most restaurant meals contain enough calories without the bread.

8. Order an entrée only. If you must have a dessert or appetizer, share!

9. As the day goes on, your need for large, high-calorie meals diminish. So, if you are out for a late dinner, stick to choices made from vegetables, salads, and lower fat protein sources (e.g., fish, chicken, extra lean cuts of red meat).

10. Always aim to leave some food on your plate—you can always take it home for tomorrow. We know it is a small demonstration, but this demonstration of discipline will help you feel like you have power over your eating habits. This sends a very clear message to yourself and to the Universe that you are serious.

"Crave the conversation, not the food!"
~Uche

SIX ESSENTIALS TO HEALTHY LIFESTYLE EATING

1. Believe that a healthy lifestyle is possible for yourself.

2. Develop a take-charge attitude. "I do what I have to do when I have to do it."

3. Create your own personal plan that works for you and your family.

4. Have positive self-talk. (It may sometimes be the only good conversation you have all day!)

5. Incorporate regular activity into your life.

6. Learn to use food as a fuel and not as an escape.

JOURNAL ACTIVITY

What changes would you like to make to your eating habits?

How does it make you feel to know you are at the fork (literally) in the road to a new way of looking at food, your body's fuel?

Breathe deeply and close your eyes and think of where your new, stronger resolve is going to take you. Write for five minutes, or on one full page in your journal, all the benefits you will enjoy with your new commitment to sound nutrition.

BEGIN TODAY

No two people are the same in terms of their exercise and nutrition needs. We have varying shapes, sizes, and metabolic rates; so don't worry if someone else's plan is not working for you! We have met hundreds of people, and every one has his or her own idea of what is the right way to go. Deep down inside, you know what you ought to be doing. The great Roman orator, Cicero said, "Nobody can give you wiser advice than yourself."

Start your investigation today and reap the benefits! Keep your eyes and ears open for sound information. And with some trial and error, you will be able to determine what is right. Waiting around for the right time to take action is simply postponing your right to enjoy good health. And once you get started and are well on your way, you'll probably ask yourself, "Why didn't I start all this sooner?"

SUGGESTED READING:

The Food Doctor by Vicki Edgson and Ian Marber
This beautiful book is full of colourful pictures and gives you the top 100 foods for enjoying a healthy life.

Intuitive Eating by Evelyn Tribole and Elyse Resch
Written by two registered dieticians, this book explains intuitive eating in an easy-to-understand style.

Fat Wars by Brad King
This is an in-depth book on performance nutrition. If you want to go to the next level, he provides great information.

Fats that Kill, Fats that Heal by Dr. Erasthmus Udo
If you are interested in learning more about the different kinds of fats and why some fats are essential, try reading this book.

Optimum Sports Nutrition by Dr. Michael Colgan
If you want to know about specific athletic nutrition, we recommend this comprehensive book.

"Approach the grocery store with a plan of action and a full stomach!"
~**Kary Odiatu**

CHAPTER EIGHT

SHOPPING 101

ဢ

"Three rules for grocery shopping: never go hungry, stay out of the junk food aisle, and (if you are a keener) tape a picture of one of your role models to your list!"
~Uche and Kary

"When the going gets tough, the tough go shopping."

"We laughed until we cried..."
~Kary

It's been said, "Shopping on an empty stomach is not a good idea." Well, of course Uche and I like to take everything to the extreme, so one day, after a long workout, we went grocery shopping. Just imagine, two hungry, tired athletes trying not to be forced into the arms of the "Supermarket Junk Food Section Monster." We were doing very well until we came to the frozen-food section where they keep the ice cream—my nemesis. Uche first noticed the colourful pint of Ben and Jerry's Chunky Monkey in the cart two minutes later. He picked it up and jokingly teased me for the little indiscretion as I half-heartedly ambled over to the frozen section and pretended to return the ice cream. (You see, we always aim to shop with the concept of Food for Function—this entails asking yourself, "Is this item going to bring me closer to how I want to look and feel?")

At the checkout, the Chunky Monkey mysteriously appeared from out of the cart and made its way onto the counter. Uche had his nose buried in a magazine, and I was hoping it would sneak by. Apparently, he sensed my uneasiness, and moments later, he looked up just as the lady was about to scan the Chunky Monkey—I was caught in the act! I put the ice cream back... or so he thought! We arrived home, and Uche remembered he had to exchange some Christmas lights—YES! Me and the Monkey, alone at last!

Uche returned home, and when he asked if I had managed to sneak the ice cream home, I innocently reminded him that he had made me put it back. He took a quick peek in the freezer and saw no sign of the Chunky Monkey.

A few hours later, Uche went to take out the garbage. He lifted the transparent garbage bag and saw a crumpled but distinctive Monkey's face mocking him through the plastic! He looked at me. We both started laughing. We laughed until we cried!

QUEST FOR FOOD

Thousands of years ago, people depended on crude weapons and their bare hands to obtain food. They gathered fruits, nuts, and vegetation and sometimes left for days to hunt. Cycles of famine and feasting meant that being lean was undesirable, and meal replacement shakes were nothing more than a fantasy!

Today, food gathering is no longer a life and death challenge for most North Americans. It has evolved into a psychological battle, where the combatants are instant gratification versus health consciousness. Our tools for gathering are credit cards, sport utility vehicles, shopping carts, and nerves of steel. The desire to kill has been quenched to a small flare of annoyance when the person ahead of you blocks the aisle for a few minutes while he tries to choose a box of cereal from the hundreds of available brands!

Dr. Peter J. D'Adamo, author of the bestseller *Cook Right 4 Your Type,* claims we don't have to carry a calculator and a fat or calorie counter or be a food scientist when we go to the market. By simply using very basic nutritional practices and focussing on choosing the freshest foods in their most natural forms, the whole process can be fairly painless.

DID YOU KNOW?

There are food brokers whose job is to strategically position certain brands on eye-level shelves? The four most-needed items (bread, milk, fruits, and veggies) are located in the far corners of the store, making it necessary to walk through the whole store? Talk about a conspiracy!

CREATE A STELLAR SHOPPING EXPERIENCE!

It is much easier to stay on track with your resolve if you attempt to integrate healthy living principles into every part of your day. If you make good choices at the supermarket, you know you have given yourself a head start.

✓ **Begin with the end in mind**. Keep your health and fitness goals in mind while you prepare a list of excellent food choices. Having clear intentions can streamline your fitness journey. Deepak Chopra in *The Seven Spiritual Laws of Success* discusses how focussed intentions and desires can enhance any experience. Look at shopping as a means of getting the fuel for your life's journey. This new way of looking at this often-dreaded task could empower you to make better choices.

✓ **Eat before you go**. Will you be strong in your intention if your stomach is growling and begging for attention? Food choices are markedly different with hunger lapping at your heels. That bag of cheese flavoured tacos that you bought for future company will not make it past the "front seat feeding frenzy" if you are famished.

✓ **Do not shop at the end of a stressful day**. It's very easy to justify poor choices if you are tired and in a hurry to get home. Checking labels and re-affirming your sound nutrition mission statement will be the furthest thing from your mind! Coaching legend, Vince Lombardi said, "Fatigue makes cowards of us all."

✓ **Synergize the experience!** Shop with someone else who also has similar sound nutritional goals. When two people shop together, they can help keep each other on track.

EIGHT IN-STORE STRATEGIES

"I soon realized Uche had some kind of
abundance shopping disorder."
~Kary

I'll never forget the first grocery shopping experience I had with my new husband. My mother did all of the shopping when I was a child, so I was surprised when Uche said he would like for us to shop together. I tentatively agreed, thinking it would go by much faster than if I had to do it alone—was I in for a shock!

With three growing boys in the family, they never seemed to be able to keep the fridge full for any length of time. Uche's mother later told me Uche went as far as counting the grapes to make sure he got his fair share!

We entered the store, and I soon realized Uche had some kind of abundance shopping disorder. He insisted on stockpiling everything from canned tuna to bread. We could barely push the loaded cart, and my mental calculator was over-heating. The scary part was that we had four more aisles left to go! We finally made it to the checkout where Uche amazed the clerk when he asked for forty-two grocery bags! I had never seen anything like it—I couldn't wait to go home and call to my mother to talk about this strange behaviour!

Maybe I had discovered why husbands don't usually do the shopping—their wives won't allow it! The bill came to a whopping $310.00!!! I found myself telling the clerk that we had six kids at home! Uche seemed very content and muttered that we would not have to shop for months. I didn't have the heart to remind him about expiration dates and rotten fruits and veggies!

Susan Powter, author of *Food*, exclaims: **"Do not leave your mind at the cart rack!"** Store managers and food brokers have many clever marketing techniques, such as: "super-size it!" "just in time for Christmas," and "you can't get a better deal!" If you do not have an organized list and a plan of action, you can end up with a five-pound bag of candy, a five-in-one plastic bowl kit, or a scented three-wick candle in your cart!

✓ **Stick to the perimeters of the supermarket**. It is not an accident that most of the healthiest food choices (fish, poultry, lean meats, fruits, veggies, eggs, and soy milk, for example) are tucked away on the outskirts of the store requiring a walk through the other aisles. By the time you have walked around the store, you will have been tempted to purchase a few items not on your list.

✓ **Read labels.** It is an enlightening experience when you find out what you are putting into your body. Studies have shown that people who read the labels on food packages are more likely to make healthier food choices. Here are a few common words used on food packaging:
  • Low fat: A product that has three or less grams of fat per serving. (Remember, *there may be more than one serving in a package!*)
  • No added sugar: This does not necessarily mean sugar free. It simply means it is processed without adding additional sugar.
  • Lite: Items that contain one-third less calories than the original item. (Not necessarily low fat.)

✓ **Fresh is best**—Canned foods have lost some of their nutrient content due to the high heat and pressure they are subjected to in the canning process. These items are usually higher in salt as well. However, nothing can beat the convenience and variety offered at the speed of a can opener! Rinsing canned foods before consuming them will remove much of the sodium.

✓ **Live foods are an essential part of a nutritious diet**. When choosing fresh fruits and vegetables, look for brightly coloured items with little or no bruising or marking. Check for firmness, and do not be scared to ask when the next shipment of fresh produce is expected. Most stores have a specified day of the week when they receive their produce. It's smart to shop within the next day or two, so you get the best quality and variety.

✓ **Choose lean ground beef** whenever possible, or try substituting lean ground turkey for beef. Another technique to avoid saturated fat is to use half meat and half dried (cooked) beans in recipes such as lasagne.

✓ **Be careful at the checkout counter**. These areas are geared for impulse buying. There has been much research on buying habits. They then use this knowledge when they set up the counters with their inviting displays of candies and other treats.

✓ **Beware of the fat-free foods**. A lot of fat-free foods are about the same amount of calories as their regular counterparts. Many of them contain even more processed chemical components and are high in sugar. It is easy to be misled into thinking fat-free foods are healthy.

ADVANCED FITNESS SHOPPING STRATEGIES

✓ **Try organically grown fruits and vegetables**. These items may cost a little more, but they will taste better and are healthier for you. If organically grown produce is not a possibility for you, then you can reduce your exposure to chemicals by washing the fruits or vegetables.

✓ **Free-range meat choices** can greatly reduce the amount of animal fat you consume if you eat meat. These meats are from animals raised with less additives to their diets. The taste may seem a little less flavourful without the high fat content, but the flesh of the animals is leaner, and the texture and colour will be richer.

✓ **Try something new**. Don't bury your head in the sand: ostrich meat has less fat than commercially raised lamb, beef, chicken, turkey, or pork. It also has fewer calories, less cholesterol, and the same amount of protein per serving. It costs more per pound than beef, but the fact that it has no bones or fat makes the price worth it. Did you know ostrich cooks in one half the time compared to beef and does not shrink unless overcooked?

✓ **Don't hesitate to tell your grocery managers that you are interested in organic and free-range foods**. They will be pleased to stock these items if they know that consumers are looking for them! Just think, you are not only taking charge of your own health but you are helping others as well.

✓ **Have fun**! Listen to a good audio-book while you're shopping. Smile at other shoppers. Joke around with the clerks. This seemingly mundane task can be a blast if you are open to enjoying the experience. C'mon give it a try!

DID YOU KNOW?

No time for shopping or cooking? The answer may be a phone call away! We recently heard about a business that will shop for and prepare meals for you according to your likes, dislikes, and health goals. Sounds like a great idea, but remember, no amount of money can buy the discipline to eat only the food that is prepared!

We no longer need a sword or a club to get a meal. But there's still the struggle of making nutritious choices when faced with the thousands of claims and guarantees like: low fat, gluten free, calorie reduced, lactose reduced, aspartame free, and organically grown. Our advice: If you can't pronounce an ingredient, or if the list says, "continued on the next side," then back away slowly, with your hands on your cart!

In all seriousness, replace your shopping frustrations with fascination. With some research and an open mind, you can become the captain of your body and the master of your soul! The key appears to be maintaining your resolve in the food-gathering stage. Now you are ready for the supermarket!

CHAPTER NINE

SUPPLEMENT SAVVY
ဆ

**"It's human behaviour to want results as fast as possible.
The first step is to learn about your body's needs—
its basic nutrition and exercise requirements.
The second step is to get started on a consistent program.
Once you have gotten some good results,
you can begin looking into supplementation."
~Kary and Uche**

We had a very full day with our lifestyle fitness presentation. We were going into overtime with some great questions on eating and incorporating exercise into an executive schedule. It was very rewarding to see the participants getting inspired to take their fitness to the next level.

One person stood up and asked the question, "How can I speed up the process?"

"There are many ways to get more out of your exercise program," we replied. Just as we started to explain sets and reps and increases in intensity, we were interrupted...

"No, I mean what would you recommend I TAKE to get there faster?" he asked.

FIRST THINGS FIRST

What is the most confusing topic on the planet? Some think the World Wide Web. Others might say, "The stock market." We would answer, "The supplement section of the supermarket." The shelves are loaded with hundreds of colourful containers filled with powders, pills, capsules, and liquids. To the uninformed, novice health enthusiast, it looks overwhelming. Even to the experienced athlete, it can be confusing!

Many people think health and fitness can be bought in a pill. Our response is always: For optimum health, you must first maximize your nourishment from food sources by making the correct quantity and quality choices from the basic food groups. Secondly, daily exercise that incorporates cardiovascular activity and resistance training is essential.

"Intense workouts that involve weight training
and aerobics increase your nutritional requirements . . .
However, vitamin and mineral supplements should not replace food.
You should be eating properly, and then add supplements."
~John Parrillo, leading sports nutritionist

WHAT EXACTLY ARE SUPPLEMENTS?

A supplement may be defined as any mineral, vitamin, amino acid, herb, or dietary substance used to increase total nutrient intake. As you can see, this definition includes a wide range of products. Our focus in this chapter is to increase your awareness about supplements and show how they could possibly help take your health and fitness to the next level.

HOW DO YOU KNOW IF YOU NEED SUPPLEMENTS?

Many people don't eat a balanced diet and do not meet all the RDA's (recommended daily allowances) for nutrients. There are many signs that something may be missing from your diet: Are your energy levels low? Is your hair dry and brittle? Do you have trouble sleeping at night? Are you frequently ill? If you have answered "Yes" to any of these questions, you may want to ask your health-care practitioner for help. They may refer you to a registered dietician.

A registered dietician can help you find out what your caloric requirements are. The amounts of the different nutrients needed by a person are influenced by body size, age, sex, environment, activity level, and current nutritional status. One or two hours of consultation could pay off handsomely. Your present nutritional practices would be analyzed and recommendations made to take your health to the next level. If you think a fee of approximately $60 an hour may be too much to invest in your health, compare it to the cost of a long-term illness.

A registered dietician is someone who has received extensive schooling in the area of food and nutrition. It is important to find someone who you are comfortable with and who is knowledgeable. If you are an athlete, then you will definitely want to find someone who has a background in dealing with sports nutrition. We recommend you go to one based on a referral from a trusted source (e.g., your doctor, chiropractor, physiotherapist, etc.).

You can also do some investigating on your own. There are many great books on the market about nutrition. You can visit your local library or bookstore to begin your search. The internet is also a fantastic resource. But, there's loads of information; that's why it's easy to become overwhelmed. To attempt to find the one source to answer all your questions would be a monumental task. Look for basic information that is backed by reputable sources (university studies, health-care practitioners, registered dieticians, etc.).

Once you TAKE ACTION and begin your investigation, you will increase your nutrition and supplement vocabulary. It is very empowering to know some of the terms in the world of nutrition. Knowledge builds on itself, and after a while, you will feel less anxiety in the supermarket looking at the shelves of nutritional products.

SEVEN REASONS TO USE SUPPLEMENTS:

1. To eliminate nutritional deficiencies. Everyone ought to eat the best quality food available. However, with the heavy refinement and processing of our food and its refrigeration and storage, nutrients are leached out every step of the way. Depletion of the nutrient value in North America's soil has a domino effect on the foods that reach the supermarket. Over-farming, excessive fertilization, and decreased crop rotation has also led to lower nutrient values.

2. To get enough vitamins and minerals for our unique needs. Our nutritional needs are not the same—it's naïve to take the recommended dose of any vitamin or supplement and assume you're getting enough for your own health benefits. Some of us may require more, some less. Only through careful study and consultation with your health-care practitioner can you determine if you are meeting your own needs.

3. To fight free radicals. Some supplements have an antioxidant effect. This means they counteract the damage done to the body by environmental pollutants (such as smog and cigarette smoke) and by the by-products of metabolic processes (the effects of stress and even exercise).

4. To decrease the effects of aging on the body. Researchers have shown many degenerative diseases are related to aging. Antioxidants may help to combat these effects.

5. To increase energy levels. Vitamins and other nutrients are necessary for the energy-producing reactions in the human cell. Most of these needs can be met with food. Depending on individual needs, supplementation may be necessary.

6. To reduce the risk of illness. It has been shown that certain supplements may help reduce the risk and help us fight specific diseases. Even though it is always best to consult and work with a qualified physician when combating disease, another adjunct is nutritional therapy. Vitamin E supplements (400 to 800 I.U. daily) have been shown in research to reduce the risk for heart attack.

7. To assist elite athletes in getting all their protein needs met without having to eat enormous amounts of food. There are also supplements available to assist athletes who are looking to go to the next level in their sport. There are numerous performance-enhancing sports supplements that have been shown to be safe and effective in enabling athletes to perform better.

> *"I made major progress in the next few months*
> *of my training program."*
> *~Kary*

I had hit a plateau in my training. I was not recuperating after workouts, my hair and skin were dry, and my nails were brittle. I hired a new trainer, and after examining my diet and training program, he noticed I was not eating enough food to support the amount of training I was doing. More importantly, he saw I had fallen into the trap that many athletic women do—I was eating a diet extremely low in essential fats. He increased my daily caloric intake with healthy food choices from the four food groups and recommended I start supplementing my diet with flaxseed oil and antioxidants like Vitamins C and E.

I agreed and noticed a major difference in my recovery from training right away. I made major progress in the next few months of my training program. At the next visit to my hairdresser, she commented on how healthy and soft my hair was!

GREATER RESULTS

One rule we like to follow is to add only one new supplement at a time to our nutritional regimen. This way we can determine if there are any positive, noticeable benefits. Or, undesirable side effects. Even though many products are called "all natural," there can be ingredients that may have an adverse effect on your system but, it's ironic that supplements are under so much scrutiny when every year thousands of people who don't use them, die prematurely from misusing food (e.g., obesity related diseases).

On a positive note, supplements can become an important part of the daily ritual of self-care. Taking supplements at the same time every day can reinforce your new resolve. By continually making a commitment to improvement, you can make small advances in your nutritional program that could take you to a new level each time.

One of the most powerful impacts of supplements is the psychological effect of doing a little more than the average person. When you know you have spent some time, energy, and money on achieving your fitness goals, you are more likely to take your efforts seriously.

It's a daily reminder that you are taking care of that beautiful vessel—your body. It's so incredible to feel that you're going in the right direction on a daily basis. You know you're dotting the i's and crossing the t's along the way.

So in the morning or evening, whenever you take your supplements, you are reaffirming your commitment to your renewed lifelong decision to take excellent care of your body. You don't have to wash your car or vacuum out the inside to make it run better. But, you can bet that the driver that does is also doing the other things, like changing the oil and getting regular tune-ups.

"My mother's early attention and encouragement
to certain food supplements started my interest
in this area."
~Uche

I remember being given cod liver oil by my mother when I was very young. It's funny now to think back and remember the disgusted look on my brothers and sisters' faces when we knew it was TIME.

My mother would bring out this large, funny-looking silver spoon after breakfast. Because of the size of the spoon, we were never quite able to get the entire amount of the thick, room temperature oil into our mouths. The result? Whoever went last would often have to also swallow what the others were unable to. There was always the inner conflict, "Should I be the first in line or the last?"

Well, looking back with what I know now about essential fats (omega-3's and omega-6's), our mother was right on track and a great role model. If you were to take a peek into one of our kitchen cupboards today, you would see the influence of my mother's early guidance.

HOW TO GET ON THE PATH

We did not provide an exhaustive list of supplements for you to read through. Our objective was to stir a desire on your part to take ownership for your health, to do some investigation on your own, and make the commitment to take your health and fitness to the next level.

There is no magic elixir for excellent health. No amount of vitamins, herbs, or minerals can replace good old-fashioned exercise and a balanced diet. But, they definitely have their place in today's world.

"If you're deficient in one or more nutrients,
it's quite possible your body may not be able to
build muscle and burn fat properly."
~Bill Phillips

SUGGESTED READING:

Nutrition Almanac, 2nd Edition by J. D. Kirchmann with L. Dunne
This best-selling book is easy to read. It starts with the basics in nutrition and goes into many of the supplements available. It also lists many common health ailments and the dietary and supplement ways to assist in their treatment. This is one of the first books Uche's mother had in their house when he was growing up.

Sports Supplement Review, 4th Issue by Vince Andrich
This is an excellent review of all the available supplements on the market. If you are interested in performance supplements, it is a very good source of information.

"The act of exercising creates energy, and as you create energy you give your body vitality. And if you have vitality, you look good."
~David Patchell-Evans

CHAPTER TEN

MOVE IT OR LOSE IT!
&

"To be alive is to be moving.
Inhibit the movement and you create illness.
To block movement is to block change.
The moving body freely channels the energy of life."
~John Travis and Regina Sara Ryan

"When you gain control of your body,
you gain control of your life."
~Bill Phillips, author of Body-*for*-LIFE

ARE YOU SUFFERING FROM HYPO KINESIS?

Hypo kinesis (hypo: under or less, kinesis: motion or activity) is a condition that affects millions of North Americans who do not make time for regular exercise. It has a ripple effect in many areas – how you feel, how you look, and how you perform daily tasks. Ten early warning signs are:

- Lack of ability to concentrate.
- Difficulty sleeping.
- Difficulty waking up.
- Feeling rundown.
- Frequent colds.
- Premature aging.
- Feeling like life is passing you by.
- Increased bodyweight.
- Getting winded walking up a flight of stairs.
- Getting winded walking down a flight of stairs (yikes!).

People often associate the word exercise with sacrifice and pain. The minute they even hear the word, they conjure up images of spending less time with their family and friends, giving up freedom, and spending incredible amounts of money on gym memberships, workout wear, and personal trainers. Many people have an *all-or-nothing* attitude that immobilizes them or postpones their movement toward health and happiness. These thinking patterns are usually strongly rooted and challenging to change.

DID YOU KNOW?

You will lose one pound of muscle every two years if you don't perform some form of resistance or weight training. Muscles get smaller when they're not stimulated. (They do not turn into fat!)

This can have a grave impact on your physical appearance. Your weight may be close to what it was ten years ago, but you may look very different.

When you have less muscle, you burn fewer calories, which will cause an increase in fat stores if your diet or activity level is not modified. Five pounds of bodyfat takes up a lot more space than five pounds of muscle! This often shows up as a "spare tire" around the abdomen or "saddlebags" on the hips.

Postponing participation in an activity that could enhance the quality of your life seems crazy, doesn't it? Waiting for that perfect time to get going is postponing enjoyment! Realistically, the chances of the perfect time arriving are pretty slim—even nonexistent.

We have a theory… the best time to get started was ten years ago. The next best time is right NOW!

FOR THE LOVE OF IT

"Movement is the essence of life. Movement is also an integral part of love, as love is always growing, moving, expanding. Love, like life, is a creative force. So why not actively participate In your relationship as you would in a sport or physical activity? As we move through our lives, we tend to move less and less. As we become adults, we seek to leave behind the things of childhood. What we've forgotten is that the playfulness of childhood is life affirming, while many of the attitudes of adulthood are deadening."
~Greg Godek (from his book *Love*)

What's love got to do with it? Excellent question. We're thrilled you asked. You see, many people attempt to get in shape for short-term, ego-bound reasons. They want to look great for some special event. They want to lose 10 pounds, even if it's going to kill them. And why?

"Summer is four weeks away."

"My thirtieth birthday is next week."

"My best friend just lost 10 pounds."

"I just made a bet with my co-worker."

"I just lost a bet with my co-worker."

How about this one: "It's my high school reunion next month." Hey, most of us know people who have thrown themselves into a Herculean workout and starvation diet to get themselves into that small dress or suit. Pure enjoyment is rarely woven into such an extreme regimen. These intense efforts may bring some immediate resuls – that's what makes them attractive. However, they aren't maintainable. It's like cramming all night for the big exam. Sure, you might pass, but the knowledge will not be retained. Short-term, ego-driven goals do not lead to lifetime habits or results.

Weak reasons like, "What will they think of me?" do not make for lasting change. The return to inactivity and past vices is inevitable. And the cycle begins again. This roller-coaster effort only perpetuates self-destructive behaviour and low self-esteem.

We encourage you to understand that there are many more powerful reasons to begin an exercise program than those mentioned above. Powerful reasons will lead to lifetime habits and results!

TEN REASONS TO GET STARTED

1. Regular exercise is one of the best things you can do to keep bodyfat at a healthy level. We have a natural tendency to store fat. One theory explains that people accumulated fat in preparation for famines over the early part of human history. Fortunately, we can fool this survival mechanism by staying active. Daily activity tells our cells that there will be a constant supply of nutrients. The cells get the message, metabolism stays high, and food gets used for fuel efficiently. Did you know that your metabolic furnace is set higher for up to ten hours after resistance training? The benefit? Calories get burned more efficiently during that time.

2.   Exercise improves mental acuity. Your blood circulates better, and you breathe more deeply. This delivers stimulating oxygen to both mind and body. It's nature's anecdote to stress, anger, and frustration, which can be obstacles to thinking clearly. Some therapists include walking as part of their clients' anger-management programs.

3.   Exercise elevates mood. Endorphins get released from the brain during exercise. Endorphins, known as nature's opiates – your body's drug of choice – put you in a euphoric state. That's why you can get addicted to the way exercise makes you feel. These feelings are your body's natural rewards for making it move. Your body just knows it's the right thing to do.

4.   Movement helps you feel rejuvenated. Experts in the field report that just 10 to 15 minutes of brisk walking may provide approximately 2 hours of elevated energy levels. After a long day at work, a session of exercise could leave you feeling refreshed. You actually experience a "second wind" following exercise.

> *"We are both seeing results with our regular workouts.*
> *And by spending such peak times with my wife,*
> *I also feel closer to her."*
> *~Dr. K. Gupta*

As an emergency room doctor, my days are long and filled with intense physical, mental, and emotional demands. It would be easy to find a comfortable spot on the couch and just relax when I arrive home.

On many evenings, I look over at my wife, and it appears we're both lacking in the energy department. One of us will always say, "Okay, let's go!" It's like we both know that a good workout will give us that much needed second wind.

Going to the gym with Rishma is such a treat. You see, I look forward to seeing her, so combining the time with her and training with weights is simply fantastic."

5.   Peace of mind can be a by-product of regular exercise. When you're doing something positive for your health, it's hard to focus on negative thoughts and feelings. Experts in the field of motivation say it's psychologically impossible for your mind to hold two opposing thoughts in the same instant. Exercise can also give you a feeling of accomplishment and a sense of control, even if the rest of your life feels out of control.

6.   Stretching will increase circulation and warm joints and muscle fibres. Better flexibility and range of motion are important for everyday tasks. Have you ever seen someone who isn't flexible bend over to pick up an

object off the floor? How about watching that same person get up off a soft, comfortable chair? With a loud grunt, he or she completes the task – it almost hurts to watch.

7. Regular exercise is an admirable lifestyle habit. So if you are looking for your soul mate or new people to flock with, try your local gym or put on some cologne and go for a run! By taking care of yourself, you're indirectly saying, "I'm valuable." And the person with a good self-concept is possibly someone who's worth getting to know!

8. People who work out consistently often have healthier lifestyle practices. They're less likely to indulge in smoking, excessive drinking, or overeating. For them, it doesn't make sense to invest time and energy in exercising without dotting their i's and crossing their t's with other healthy habits. There's a domino effect; if you start an exercise program, you're likely to begin eating better. It just makes sense!

9. The body will be less prone to disease and illness. With increased circulation and oxygenation of the entire body, toxins and waste can be eliminated more efficiently. Exercise also prevents the build-up of fat and cholesterol in the arteries and decreases the chance of blood clots. Nutrients are transported efficiently to all areas of the body. The list goes on. Do you need more convincing? Think of it as an insurance plan for your body. It's one of the best investments you can make! We're talking as little as 20 minutes 3 times a week!

10. "MOTION CREATES EMOTION." If two people love each other, they can enhance their relationship by exercising and experiencing those feel-good endorphins together. Research has shown that participating in a joint physical fitness regimen is a great way to show mutual support and caring. Paul Pearsall, in *Ten Laws of Lasting Love,* shares that couples who learn to play together, stay together. He goes on to say that in play as well as sport, we open ourselves to other realities. The endorphins that are released into our bloodstreams while having fun can bring families together. We know we live in a world where we play to win. However, the magical family wins by playing.

"One person caring about another
represents life's greatest value."
~Jim Rohn

COMMON MISCONCEPTIONS ABOUT EXERCISE

I have to lose bodyfat before I get started on a resistance or weight-training program.

REALITY: Resistance training is one of the best ways to help you lose fat. When you lift weights, you can significantly increase your metabolic rate (the rate your body burns calories). When you add more muscle to your frame (or get more toned), your body requires more energy to maintain that muscle tone. Aerobic exercise can get you into a fat-burning zone for a short period of time, but adding more muscle raises your thermostat for the long haul.

I'm too tired to work out after a long day at the office.

REALITY: The hormones associated with physical activity will re-energize and re-vitalize you. Once you get yourself moving, you'll be glad you did physically and psychologically! Believe us, there are days when we don't feel like going to the gym either. And there's the occasional time when we don't go. One thing is for sure – we have never regretted going! Exercise gives you that second wind for your evening activities.

> The key is to "just do it" (like the Nike ad says!).
> It doesn't matter when. Whenever you can make time -
> before work, midday, or even late at night.

I exercise, so I can eat whatever I want.

REALITY: To maximize the full benefits of exercise, you need foods high in nutrients. Nutritional deficiencies can occur if you exercise with a depleted body. Many people start an exercise program without making any nutritional changes (or they eat even more of the wrong foods because they think they're justified with the increase in activity). And then they wonder why they don't see any results. Too often they quit their programs, chalking their weight problems up to genetics or a thyroid problem.

"I'll never look like Madonna, so why get started?"

REALITY: It's never a good idea to compare yourself to others. Why would you want to give your personal power away? The best way to challenge yourself is to set measurable, attainable goals that motivate you. Be the best YOU that you can be!

Being a woman, I'm afraid I'll get bulky if I lift weights.

REALITY: Did you know that fat takes up more space than muscle? In other words, losing fat and building muscle means that even though you may weigh the same, your problem areas will be much smaller (think of your hips and thighs). You can change your shape dramatically by adding more muscle to your shoulders and chest, creating the appearance of a smaller waist and thighs.

Muscles do not show up overnight! It's a gradual process, and you are totally in control of how big you would like them to be. Once you are satisfied with your level of muscle tone, you can then do a maintenance program. Muscles will not keep growing unless they are constantly challenged with increasing weights or intensity. You are in complete control over how developed you become. It's not as if one morning you will wake up with arms like Arnold Schwarzenegger dangling from your shoulders!

"Now, at age 32, I feel better about myself than ever before!"
~Kary

I have seen my body go through a miraculous transformation since I began weight training in my early 20's. I once described myself as pear shaped – with more fat on my thighs and hips and not enough muscle tone on my chest, back, shoulders, and arms. You could not pay me to wear tights that would emphasize my "saddlebags."

I now train extremely hard with heavy weights and follow a disciplined yet balanced nutrition program. I do not feel bulky with my muscularity; I feel sleek, strong, and toned. I am in control of how much muscle I choose to carry – I can increase it or decrease it by manipulating my exercise program and nutritional intake. Now, at age 32, I feel better about myself than ever before!

DID YOU KNOW?

Legendary beauty Marilyn Monroe lifted weights but would never let on about it for fear of society's condemnation of it? Marilyn was definitely ahead of her time; she knew resistance training would give her many benefits.

I'm too old to make any significant changes with my body.

REALITY: At about the age of 25, your muscle mass starts to slowly decrease and your bodyfat stores increase if you do not add resistance training and proper nutrition and cardiovascular training to your life. With this decrease in muscle, we become fragile, weak, and prone to injury. Bill Phillips mentions in his book, Body-*for*-LIFE, that a study from Tufts University showed that a 3-times-per-week weight-training program done with men between the ages of 60 to 72 caused an increase in flexibility and strength of up to 200%. The best thing is that anyone can start weight training today and reap the rewards!

I don't have enough time to work out.

REALITY: It is definitely possible to make gains with short, intense workouts. There's no need for marathon sessions to enjoy the rewards of exercise. Even 15 minutes done regularly during your lunch hour will yield results!

DID YOU KNOW?

Building your back muscles with resistance training helps you in many other areas aside from looking good at the beach. Working on those hard-to-see muscles will make you stronger in every task—gardening, housekeeping, playing with the kids, etc. Another bonus is better posture, which helps you look more attractive and protects your spine from injury.

You have to lift weights every day to gain muscle.

REALITY: Muscles are broken down during exercise. It is the *rest time* following the workout when the body repairs the muscle tissue, making it even stronger and bigger. If you are not giving your body enough rest/recovery/re-growth time, you won't experience gains in strength or size. The body part that has been trained requires about 48 hours to recover properly.

There are many different ways to schedule your workouts in a week to maximize your training. There are many programs that will work: the key is to find something you enjoy and can implement into your life. Pick one to start, and then experiment with others and make your own choices. Again, this is where a personal trainer or your own research will be of value. The key is to start now!

> *"I'm a busy guy who has made exercise*
> *a ritual part of my life."*
> *~Uche*

I train with weights three to four times per week and spend about one hour at the gym per session. These weight-training sessions include a 5- to 10-minute warm-up on a bike, weights, and a warm-down/flexibility session of about 5 minutes at the end. I do a 20-minute cycle on our exercise bike at home while I watch TV or read a book every other day. The most time I spend exercising in any one day is about one hour! This means there's lots of time for the other things I enjoy in life.

TEN STEPS TO EXERCISE SUCCESS

Get your physician's approval before starting any physical fitness program.

1. Make a public statement to key people in your life about your goals for the future. In the beginning, you may not be comfortable sharing with anyone. That's OK! You may want to think of yourself working on your own special project – YOU. There may come a time when sharing is okay. It all depends on the people you have in your life. Be careful that you share with people who will support you, not criticize or ridicule you. A new goal is like a fragile flower, which needs support and nurturing. There's nothing like having people in your life who want the best for you and who support you unconditionally!

2. Set realistic deadlines for the accomplishment of your goals. Deadlines create a sense of urgency. If you don't put a timeline on fulfilling your fitness desires, they will remain unfulfilled dreams. We used the term realistic, so you wouldn't set yourself up for failure with deadlines that require Herculean efforts. Remember to enjoy the journey!

3. Keep an exercise log and record your efforts and improvements. This can be highly motivating and also excellent for reviewing your progress and setting new goals.

4. Form a clear picture of your lifelong goals for fitness. Try this as you awaken in the morning, before you get out of bed. At this time, your mind is very open to suggestion. Create mental pictures of yourself or your family reaping the benefits of fitness. This little exercise will open the door to a whole new level of success. This strategy can assist you in manifesting your goals and has been recognized by many success philosophers throughout recorded history (Benjamin Franklin, Napoleon Hill, Wayne Dyer, Anthony Robbins, and Andrew Carnegie, to name a few).
    Visualization is a powerful process that all successful people use. If you have a hard time using your imagination, buy yourself a scrapbook. Fill it with pictures of people who are doing the things you want to do. Cut out pictures from fitness magazines of physiques that inspire you. Or you could use pictures of yourself at a time when you felt healthy and full of life.

5. Face your fears! Fears can be squashed with action! The first taste of freedom will come when you face something you have put off because of some self-imposed fear or limitation. Many of us have been immobilized because we are afraid to be judged or to look

like a beginner. There is a whole other world outside the boundary of a personal fear. Conquering it would lead to unbelievably liberating levels of enjoyment or "fulthrillment" as author Mark Victor Hansen says.

DID YOU KNOW?
There is a bright side to being a beginner! When you are new to a sport or activity, you will actually burn more calories per hour during that activity than someone who is proficient at it. In the beginning, you need to expend a lot of effort and make more attempts to achieve the desired results (e.g., a beginner at golf will have to take many more strokes than a professional).

---

6. Give yourself some variety – try walking, running, cycling, or even indoor rock climbing to put some spice into your training program. Cross training prevents overuse injuries and boredom and provides for overall development. The key is to put an increased demand on your heart and lungs and use the large muscle groups of the body in a variety of ways.

7. Choose a time to exercise and stick to it, so you can have a scheduled routine. By making it a "must" instead of a "should," you feel more committed to do what you say. In the beginning of your program, it's very important to honour your commitment. Missing just one session can lead to many more missed workouts.

8. Perform a warm-up to clear your mind and focus on the upcoming workout and a cool-down to reflect on your training and goals. These are easy steps to skip, but the best athletes in the world manage to do them every time.

9. Make sure your goals are realistic or attainable. Start slowly – two or three times per week is achievable and maintainable. It would be unrealistic to train for a full marathon in 3 months if you were never a runner. Enthusiasm is excellent. But doing too much too soon will lead to burn out or injury.

10. Make a commitment to celebrate your victory over complacency every time you work out. People have a tendency to celebrate only large goals or milestones, like losing 20 pounds or winning a competition. The human psyche loves reinforcement. Without rewards along the way, it's very easy to become disillusioned and discouraged.

"Good people strengthen themselves ceaselessly."
~Confucius

JOURNAL ACTIVITY

Name three things you are committed to achieving with your new exercise program:

1.

2.

3.

What are the benefits to you if these goals are achieved? What kind of life will you be living?

Who else would benefit from these results?

What is one step you can take today?

> "Your talent determines what you can do.
> Your motivation determines how much you are willing to do.
> Your attitude determines how well you do it."
> ~Lou Holtz, author of *Winning Every Day*

HOW TO KEEP THE NEW WHEEL TURNING

The *Journal of Sports Medicine and Physical Fitness* reported that over half of all men and 65% of women who begin a regular exercise and nutrition program drop out within 3 months. To avoid being a statistic, you can bolster yourself by trying the following:

1. Be a lifelong student. Learn about exercise (techniques and principles) and nutrition. Get a subscription to an exercise magazine, such as *Muscle and Fitness, Muscle and Fitness Hers, Men's Health, Men's Fitness, Oxygen, Shape,* or *Fitness.* There are also many videos and books available.

2. Hire a trainer – a little research and checking references can lead you in the right direction.

3. Observe and talk to others who have made transformations and maintained them. Their testimonies will inspire you and give you confidence that it can be done.

4. Work out with a partner and share the experience. You will be less likely to skip workouts if someone else is depending on you to be there.

THE END RESULT

Exercise time can become one of your favourite times of day. Taking action every day on the path to health feels *soooo* satisfying. Have we stirred you into thinking about getting started? There's no other investment that will give you as much return as physical fitness. There is no property or stock that can make you feel the way a healthy body can.

There is a ripple effect that comes with a commitment to an exercise program. You will be inspired to drink more water, to eat better, to begin writing your thoughts in a journal, and to share your experiences with the important people in your life.

A disciplined self-action plan exercises more than just muscles. Doing what you have to do when you have to do it is great for your psyche. The early return on this new behaviour is great. The long-term return is fantastic!

So, walk away from the crowd and become part of the group that's enjoying the good life. The real key to living a life of happiness is the continuous movement toward your dreams and goals. Benjamin Disraeli explains it this way: "The secret of success is constancy of purpose."

"Anytime you are living in the present and consciously improving your situation, you will have boundless energy, mental acuity, and joy."
~Kary

SUGGESTED READING:

Living the Good Life by David Patchell-Evans
This five-time Canadian rowing champion recounts his own personal story and gives inspiring tips on diet and exercise. The message is simple—maybe not everyone can be an athlete, but everyone can be fit!

Body-for-LIFE by Bill Phillips
If you're looking for a program you can use to make gains and implement easily into your daily life, we recommend you read Body-*for*-LIFE by Bill Phillips. His program and exercise information are easy to read and understand. The book also contains pictures of the exercises, nutrition advice, and inspiration. It is a great tool for a lifetime of fitness.

"Take your fitness resolve with you on the road. Staying true to your goals will re-affirm your commitment."
~Kary & Uche Odiatu

CHAPTER ELEVEN

HEALTHY LIFESTYLE ON THE ROAD
ಇಲ

**"Twenty years from now you will be more disappointed
by the things that you didn't do than by the things you did do.
So throw off the bowlines. Sail away from the safe harbor.
Catch the trade winds in your sail. Explore, dream, discover."
~Mark Twain**

A GLOBAL LIFESTYLE

People today are traveling with increasing frequency and urgency. They want a full experience and the opportunity to use all of their senses. Scenes of the pyramids of Gaza, the Eiffel Tower, and the other wonders of our world entice us to the many travel agencies that can provide the best experience to suit our desires. The culinary delights of different destinations tempt us into trying new foods.

Is it possible to stick to a health and fitness regimen when traveling? We say, "Of course!" But, we didn't say it was easy. People are always a little intrigued when they discover that we maintain our fitness strategies when we travel. Most believe our commitment must just be super strong. Sure it's strong. But the truth is: if we can do it, anyone can.

A vacation or business trip *can* include fitness and sound nutrition. A vacation is also a perfect opportunity to try some new activities; they may even last a lifetime – long after your tan wears off. The habit of training at a gym or going for evening walks could possibly be the greatest souvenir to bring home with you!

William James, the father of psychology, claimed that if we seize every opportunity to act on our resolutions, we increase the likelihood of attaining our goals. As a result, everyone will be amazed and surprised when you return from your trip possibly in better shape than when you left!

STAYING FIT ON THE TRIP!

All it takes is a little discipline, a firm commitment, and some effective planning to start linking positive habits to your travels. We know that can be easier said then done. Being away from home base, you'll encounter new challenges with regard to your regular food choices. But why not enjoy the local cuisine and see if you can still practice sound nutrition?

The key to enjoying the whole process is to do your best. That's all you can ask of yourself. If you spend the entire week lounging around drinking Mai Tai's and never hit the swimming pool, is that the end of the world? No. However, feeling guilty about it and beating yourself up when you get home are not very good habits to get into.

The following practices repeated often enough will become habits that will help you feel and look great during and after your next trip.

AFFIRMATION—Declare daily the importance of staying true to your nutritional goals before you leave. Remind yourself of the hard work and effort you have put toward your fitness so far. Decide ahead that you will follow sound nutritional practices 90% of the time, so you will be able to enjoy the occasional indulgence. And if you let some of your supportive travel pals or your family in on your resolve, they can become co-conspirators in your fitness quest.

HYDRATE—Drink plenty of water before you head out. A well-hydrated body is less prone to jet lag, water retention, and headaches. Don't forget to bring drinking water on the plane: that shot glass of water you get from the flight attendant is barely enough to wet your whistle! Remember that caffeine and alcoholic beverages have a diuretic effect that will only add to your feelings of malaise.

PACK SNACKS—Some of the downsides of traveling include missed flights, long waits, delays, and expensive airport food. There are many tasty, healthy snacks that are easy to pack. We always travel with a supply of protein bars, rice cakes, fruit, and meal-replacement shakes. These are food items that can be eaten anywhere: in a long line-up rescheduling a flight, waiting for the next flight in an airport lounge, or in a taxi on the way to your hotel. This helps us avoid the roller coaster ride of starving and then overeating.

PRE-ORDER—Airlines now offer a variety of special menus that can be pre-ordered through your travel agent. You can request meals that are low in fat, gluten free, kosher, cholesterol free, or vegetarian, etc. Save those fancy dinners for the nice restaurants at your destination. (A little bonus for special ordering: you're often served before everyone else!)

SUPERMARKET—One of your first destinations upon arrival should be a local grocery store where you can stock up on some food items for the hotel room. Excellent choices are bagels, apples, rice cakes, bananas, nuts, rye bread, tuna, and salmon (buy the cans with the pull-off lids if you forgot a can opener). Buy instant oatmeal to prepare in the room using hot water from the coffee maker or your own small electric kettle. This idea will save you from the late night "hotel vending-machine munchies." Plus, having a quick breakfast in your room means more time for sightseeing!

TRAIN—Try to book a hotel that has an onsite facility or a gym nearby. Even a half hour workout done two or three times during the vacation will refresh you and help to maintain your current fitness level.

"It was a great way to make some new friends!"
~Uche

We were in Australia for the World Amateur Fitness Championships in 1999. Kary needed to practice her routine, so we decided to venture out and leave the predictability of the hotel's fitness centre. We have found over the years that a local gym is the perfect place to meet people who live in the area. We were not disappointed at the Coogee Beach gym. We met some awesome people who gave us real insight into the Australian lifestyle. They told us things to do and see that were not on the "tourist attractions" list at the hotel.

RESTAURANT—You can still eat a very healthy meal at a restaurant. Most restaurants will prepare food especially for you if you just ask. Our favourite restaurant choices are baked potatoes, skinless chicken breasts, lean cuts of meat, steamed veggies, whole-wheat pancakes (ask for fruit instead of butter and syrup), brown or wild rice, eggs (egg beaters or egg whites only), and salads. Even fast-food restaurants have some healthier choices and will prepare food without the extra sauces, butter, and mayo.

Again the concept we champion is to eat healthy approximately 90% of the time. This 90/10 ratio maintains sanity and allows for treats at birthday parties, weddings, and special nights out with friends and family.

In 1991, USA General Schwarzkopf didn't head into Iraq to fight Saddam Hussein without a plan, saying, "Let's just wing it, guys!" He had Desert Storm. We encourage you to have a travel strategy (your own "*Dessert Storm*") so you will be able to reaffirm your commitment to good health for all your journeys.

"You are the architect of your life and you decide your destiny."
~Swami Rama

JOURNAL ACTIVITY

Write down the three strategies you would like to try on your next trip:

1.

2.

3.

CHAPTER TWELVE

FUTURE FIT
ଔ

"Let others lead small lives, but not you. Let others argue over small things, but not you. Let others cry over small hurts, but not you. Let others leave their future in someone else's hands, but not you."
~Jim Rohn

"People say I'm still around because I have a lot of heart, but I know all the heart in the world couldn't have helped me if I weren't physically fit."
~Jimmy Connors, former tennis sensation

"You can affect the aging process through choices."
~David Kern, N.D., naturopathic physician

REINVENTION AS AN OPTION

"I'm afraid of losing my independence. I feel lonely without my spouse. Many of my friends have passed on, the world is moving too quickly, and I miss the way things used to be. I don't want to live in a nursing home. My favourite foods hurt my stomach; my body just won't cooperate with me any more. I am tired, weak, and sore. I want to see my children and grandchildren more often, but I'm afraid to travel alone."
~Anonymous

The above story is a tough one to read. But, fortunately, aging does not have to be this way. Instead of conforming to preconceived notions of old age; seniors have the option of re-inventing themselves. Today's seniors are the pioneers of the new aging: they are going to university, they are working in and out of their homes, and they are discovering new hobbies.

If you don't renovate, things deteriorate!

The ideas of renewal and personal development after 55 were not so important 100 years ago because people, on average, did not live much past 55! Now we are living well into our 80's and beyond. Remember that the retirement age of 65 was chosen many years ago when life expectancy was much shorter!

In the new millennium, we have many tools at our disposal to live long and healthy lives. We have advanced medical technology. The number of naturopaths, osteopaths, massage therapists, chiropractors, and acupuncturists is growing rapidly. We have greater access to information: specialty magazines, the World Wide Web, and hundreds of channels on TV are spewing out information on health and vitality faster than we can keep up with it!

DID YOU KNOW?

Steven Austad of the University of Idaho says that the first person to reach 150 years of age may be alive as you are reading this book. (Kary thinks she *is* that person!) Human beings are living longer than ever as more and more research is being done on the topic.

RE-INVENTION AT ITS FINEST!

The term mid-life crisis is only a modern-day phenomenon. Life is no longer about survival; our society values contribution, personal fulfillment, and achievement. People have the luxury of more leisure time to think and ponder when they reach their 40's and 50's. For some, pondering may lead to panicking. They wake up one day and do a little review of all their choices. And they wonder why they haven't accomplished more.

For some people, growing older doesn't mean living with lower expectations. They look to the future with anticipation versus fear. If you look, you can find people in your life that exemplify the possibility that growing older does not necessarily mean failing health and reduced vitality – people who are reinventing themselves by trying new things and keeping their outlook fresh. If you can't think of any, read some biographies or watch Biography on the Arts and Entertainment Channel.

There are many well-known people in their 50's, 60's and 70's maintaining active careers and staying fresh with new projects: Ted Turner, Sylvester Stallone, Goldie Hawn, Cher, Kirk Douglas, Sophia Loren, and Arnold Schwarzenegger to list only a few.

INSPIRING PEOPLE

- Mark Victor Hansen (co-author of *Chicken Soup for the Soul*) tells a story of a 65-year-old retired postal worker who created a career for himself in his own community. He began taking care of peoples' homes, plants, and pets while they were away on business or vacation. He was able to increase his business quickly with his status as a retired senior citizen. He eventually had to hire other senior citizens, and his venture became a million-dollar enterprise!

- John Glenn came out of retirement to re-enter the world of space travel at age 78.

"My view is that to sit back and let fate play its hand and never influence it is not the way man was meant to operate."
~Ex-Astronaut and U.S. Senator John Glenn

- Nobel prizewinner Albert Schweitzer took up medicine in midlife. He worked into his 80's in his famous African hospital.

- Ben and Joe Weider founded the International Federation of Bodybuilding in 1947. Today, in their 70's, they are still very active in their organization.

- Famous artist Grandma Moses took up painting in her late 70's.

- Oscar winner Shirley Maclaine trekked 500 miles in 30 days on a spiritual pilgrimage (The Camino) in Spain. Shirley is in her 60's.

- Ronald Reagan became President of the United States in his late 60's. He went on to become one of the most charismatic world leaders of the twentieth century.

- The founder of Kentucky Fried Chicken started his multi-million dollar business at 62!

- Kary's Grandma Mary maintains her own immaculate home and garden in her mid 80's. She travels once a year out to the west coast to visit other family.

- Kary's Grandpa Dan (in his late 70's) is a voracious reader, loves a good conversation, and is always creating things with his hands.

- Uche's mother started practicing Tai Chi in her 70's and now leads the class when the instructor is away. Research has shown Tai Chi can increase cardiovascular health and improve strength, balance and flexibility. (We recently overheard her saying that she has leather pants on her wish list for Christmas!)

- Uche's father, Peter (age 70) rides his bike to the gym and enjoys weight training. We love hearing from our gym manager that some weeks he is there more than we are!

- Justice Oliver Wendell Holmes was writing Supreme Court decisions at 90. When President-elect Franklin Roosevelt paid a visit to Holmes in 1933, Holmes was reading Plato in Greek. When Roosevelt asked why, the 92-year-old Holmes answered, "Why, to improve my mind."

- The great inventor Thomas Edison was busy in his lab at age 84.

- Benjamin Franklin was helping with the completion of the American Constitution at age 70.

- Mother Theresa spent most of her 87 years on the planet devoted to helping others.

- Michael Jordan (approaching 40) is playing in the NBA; Jim Cameron (late 40's) is playing professional football in the CFL. We have more and more examples of people participating in elite levels of sports well beyond their 20's.

How old would you be if you did not know how old you were?

"IT AIN'T OVER TILL IT'S OVER"

Baseball great Yogi Berra said it well. Have you ever left a baseball or football game early to beat the traffic? And then on your car radio, you heard your team made a dramatic comeback; the game went into overtime, and your team won the game? And there you were, stuck in traffic, hearing the cheering fans enjoying your team's magical moment.

How does this apply to life? Many people leave the game early. In their 50's and 60's, they start winding down – they work less, they expect less from themselves, and they stop taking care of themselves. They say: "Why bother? I have only a few good years left. It's all downhill from here."

"I am reminded on a daily basis just how immobilizing self-limiting thoughts can be."
~Uche

I am reminded on a daily basis just how immobilizing self-limiting thoughts can be. I listened to a patient in one of my dental chairs report he didn't have to take care of his teeth anymore because he's 60 now and doesn't have much time left. The irony is that in the treatment room beside us, I had a 72-year-old patient getting her teeth whitened because she wanted to freshen up her smile!

A NEW WAY OF THINKING

"I have only one wrinkle and I'm sitting on it!"
~Jeanne Calment (lived to 122 years of age)

Can we stop the aging process? Or even better, reverse it? First, we have to get away from old, fixed, stale ideas about aging. These fixed ideas can create very real limits on our expectations for our senior years. Yes, it used to be a time of ailments and limitations and old-folks homes. But now, with the knowledge and use of fitness, nutrition, and mind/body medicine, the experience of being older has radically changed.

Experts used to think that progressive muscle weakness was inevitable. They have since discovered that it is simply the result of a lack of stimulation to the muscles.

"To me, old age is always fifteen years older than I am."
~Bernard Baruch

Many people are taking their finances seriously and planning for retirement. The 10% solution for saving and investing, championed by financial advisors, seems to be the answer. But, what is the point of "Freedom 55" without being well physically, mentally, and spiritually. How can we truly enjoy the abundance that we are trying to create without taking care of ourselves?

DID YOU KNOW?
The number of centenarians is rising. A census report stated that there were 72,000 people over 100 in the USA. This number will reach almost 1 million by 2050.

FIXED BELIEFS

The power of fixed beliefs was illustrated profoundly in a university experiment where two species of fish (predator and prey) were separated in a tank by a glass wall for several weeks. The predators kept butting themselves against the wall at first, trying to get to their prey. Eventually they stopped trying, realizing that they could not cross the boundary of the glass wall. When the wall finally was removed, the fish lived out the rest of their lives without crossing the imaginary border. Like the fish with the perceived barrier, many people maintain old limiting beliefs that have outworn their use. Lives get played out without ever challenging them, and they never cross over to new territory.

You may have heard of Roger Bannister, the first person to run a mile in under four minutes. Prior to 1954, this was believed to be an impossible human feat. But Roger ignored the fixed beliefs of exercise physiologists and scientists of the day. Interestingly enough, within the first few years after Roger broke through that limit, many others repeated his performance. This story is only one of many that proves fixed beliefs can limit our physical potential!

ADDING LIFE TO YOUR YEARS

Scientists who study aging have a term called "Biomarkers." These are not body paints! These are changes like skin loosening, vision impairment, hearing fading, muscles dwindling, immunity weakening, and brain cells dying (starting at age 30 if there's no intervention).

On the other hand, Walter Bortz, M.D., a physician and author of *We Live Too Short and Die Too Long,* says the human body has real renewable qualities: by taking responsibility for ourselves, taking charge of important areas in our lives, exercising regularly, and eating with sound nutrition, we can extend our life expectancy.

"Destiny is not a matter of chance; it's a matter of choice."
~William Jennings Bryan

Ben Douglas, Ph.D., author of *Ageless: Living Younger Longer*, reports that our bodies are meant to live approximately five times the age of our sexual maturity. In other words, human bodies are designed to live around 110 years. You are *meant* to live many more years than you have been led to believe. And many of the determining factors are in your control.

HOW CAN YOU GET STARTED?

There are many healthy habits that can add years to your life: a positive attitude, increased activity, cessation of smoking, and better food choices can all affect the aging process. Dr. Thomas T. Perls and Margery H. Silver's book *Living to 100: Lessons in Living to Your Maximum Potential at Any Age* is an excellent resource for more age-defying tips. We have compiled the following tips to give you a head start on your future fitness.

- The fountain of youth is within you. We have seen people who are 70 and older taking an active role in their environment. They don't use phrases that imprison them: "My old bones." "You can't teach an old dog new tricks!" "I'm too old!" "It's all downhill from here." "I only have a few good years left, you know…" This way of life allows them to view the future with anticipation instead of frustration.

- Make yourself indispensable. By volunteering your time and energy, you can add value to any cause. It is one of the simplest ways to make a difference. It doesn't cost anything, and there are an endless number of organizations and causes that are in need of people like you.

- Creating balance in your life can help decrease stress. Chronic stress left unchecked has been related to decreased immune-system functioning, cardiovascular disease, and digestive disorders.

- Become attached to your dreams! Having projects that you are actively working on adds passion to your daily existence. Howard E. Hill, in *Energizing the 12 Powers of the Mind,* reported that having ongoing projects at any age is a definite way to escape mediocrity. We believe the rewards and benefits will ripple out to all areas of your life. There is an old saying that goes… "There is not much to do but bury a man when the last of his dreams are dead."

- Researchers have shown that our surroundings affect us. Colours, textures, brightness, open spaces… all can help shape the way we feel. Why not take charge of your environment, so it refreshes and rejuvenates you.

- Stay sexually active! Studies have shown that couples who maintain an active sex life have more emotional, mental, and physical enjoyment as they age. At a basic level, regular exercise improves physical fitness and self-esteem, and sexual functioning is related to those areas.

- Do good deeds! Operating from the goodness of your heart adds life to your years and years to your life. The bestseller *Random Acts of Kindness* tells of the karmic energy that comes as a by-product of doing good deeds for others.

- Start new projects. Putting ideas into effect and setting plans in motion can give you big reasons to get up in the morning. There is nothing like having a large to-do list to bring out the CEO in you!

- Keep your mind flexible and open. Make an effort to surround yourself with others who are open and positive. Attitudes are extremely contagious. If you regularly get together with people who discuss only tragedies in the newspaper, recent illness, and their worries, your psyche will suffer. Avoid hardening of the mental arteries!

"To be able to find joy in another's joy: that is the secret of happiness."
~George Bernanos

- Take advantage of the Law of Forgiveness in your life. In order to enjoy excellent health and peace of mind, one must be able to forgive and forget. Holding grudges may hold anyone back from ever achieving his or her true potential and ultimate joy in life.

- The overall peace of mind that comes out of quiet reflection can add great depth to your life. It is challenging for most people to make time for daily meditation and journaling practices. But consider that you may be able to share your insights and words of wisdom from your journals with your loved ones.

"We don't stop having fun when we're old;
we're old when we stop having fun."
~Anonymous

ACTION STEPS TO AGING GRACEFULLY

All the good intentions in the world won't help you unless you start putting into action some of the little things:

1. Smile more. If you frown or scowl a lot, you will create vertical wrinkles between your eyebrows. Repetitive expressions, which tell of sadness, suffering, and anger can distort the skin, leaving permanent reminders.

2. Wear a baseball cap and/or sunscreen. The sun's ultraviolet rays affect the collagen layers in our skin, causing us to look older, faster.

3. Don't follow yo-yo diets. Weight fluctuations stretch the skin, and the skin has a difficult time regaining its appearance each time the weight is lost and regained.

4.   Wear properly fitted, comfortable shoes. If you buy poor-fitting shoes or wear old, outworn ones, you will flatten your feet and cause deformities.

5.   Sleep with the back of your head on the pillow. If you sleep with the side of your face on the pillow, more wrinkles may develop on the side of the face that lies on the pillow.

6.   Limit sun exposure and keep skin moisturized. Skin begins to lose its elasticity in our 30's, and wrinkles begin to develop.

7.   Wear protection when near loud, continuous noise. Hearing naturally declines with age, but you can prevent the acceleration of this process by taking care to protect your ears if they are constantly bombarded with loud noises.

8.   Ask your optometrist about eye exercises. The eye lens stiffens with age. Dr. Deepak Chopra, in his audio-program Magical Mind Magical Body, shares with his listeners a series of eye exercises that may be used to lessen the effect of aging on the eye muscles.

9.   Take care of your teeth and gums. Did you know that the bacteria in the mouth have been implicated in certain cardiac conditions? Research has shown that by daily flossing and regular dental visits we can possibly increase our lifespan by six years.

EXERCISE ENHANCES LIFE

> **"Sometimes I have to drag my butt off the couch to get to the
> recreation centre, but I feel great when I am finished.
> I never regret going once I am done!"**
> **~Ruth Milbradt, retired teacher**

> **"Exercise, a whole-food diet, and supplements are what you need to
> avoid spending your retirement in the doctor's office."**
> **~Glenn Cassie,**
> **Director of the British Columbia Naturopathic Association**

The role of exercise is vital to aging gracefully. Basically, if you don't use it, you lose it! People who tend to have a couch potato lifestyle when they are younger often end up as mashed potatoes when they are older. Dr. Steven Lamm, author of *Younger at Last: The New World of Vitality Medicine*, reports that non-active people lose approximately one pound of muscle every two years after age twenty. Less muscle mass means less fat-burning potential, which leads to increased fat storage.

Anyone who has fixed ideas about resistance / weight training will never see the benefits of toned muscles. Many women believe they'll get bulky or manly if they train with weights, but in fact, women don't have enough of the male sex hormone, testosterone, to add large muscles to their bodies.

In reality, men and women should be more concerned about having too little muscle, rather than too much! Muscle is a very active, highly functioning tissue. When you have more muscle and less fat on your body, you have increased ability to enjoy all of life's activities.

"The more my muscles get developed, the easier it is to lift my shopping bags. More importantly, how else am I going to be able to lift my grandson? Heaven forbid if I had to carry him if there was an emergency! I have signed up for a weight-training course for seniors."
~Mary Odiatu

Without stimulation, muscles begin to shrink, and the number of muscle fibres decreases. Lifting weights or resistance training for as little as 20 minutes, 3 times per week will reverse this process. In addition, a stretching and flexibility program will allow you to stay limber, resist injury, and feel youthful. Try looking under health or fitness in the yellow pages to find information about trainers, gyms, and community clubs.

The benefits of exercise are numerous, and it is never too late to get started. In one study, 300 hospital patients (over 70 years of age) were divided into 2 groups after an extended stay. Only one of the groups was given an exercise program to follow. It was found that this group was able to go about their daily activities much better than the group that didn't follow the exercise program.

In a study where 84 individuals from 50 to 72 years of age were being treated for clinical depression, those who followed a regular aerobic exercise program showed physical benefits, and improved brain functions. If you are interested in having a stronger more powerful immune system, consistent participation in an exercise program is one of the keys. Regular exercise has positive effects on a number of medical conditions that have been associated with the elderly:

1. Lowers diabetes risk
2. Helps manage stress
3. Helps prevent osteoporosis
4. Increases good cholesterol and decreases blood pressure
5. Decreases joint stiffness and increases mobility
6. Decreases risk of many cancers
7. Helps regulate hormone levels (during menopause)
8. Increases memory and other mental abilities
9. Decreases osteoarthritis and joint pain
10. Helps control body weight

If the material in this chapter is making sense to you, then it may be a great time to go back to Chapter 3 (Set a Goal, Get a Goal). If you did not do the goal setting exercises, the perfect time is now! They are a great way to give you solid reasons to begin/continue your exercise program.

"Growing weaker is not a consequence of aging, but rather the result of not using muscles optimally."
~Dr. Steven Lamm

NUTRITION

Following sound nutritional principles is one of the easiest ways to *age-proof* yourself. But, what appears easy to do is easy not to do. The chapter "Food for Function" applies to all ages. And if its recommendations are put to use, they could help with your quest for a long and healthy life. We have compiled a list of nutritional recommendations specifically for seniors.

Remember to consult your physician before making any changes to your nutrition or supplementation program.

- Drink water to keep your kidneys in shape. Kidneys lose function naturally about one percent per year. Drinking at least six to eight glasses per day becomes even more important as we get older.

- Stay current with what's new in nutrition. There is always new literature on healthy eating and its effects on our bodies. Be a life-long learner, and stay on top of recent discoveries in the world of nutrition.

- Eat more of the top anti-cancer foods as listed in the easy-to-read book *The Food Doctor*: broccoli, cauliflower, cabbage, brown rice, Brussel sprouts, soya, garlic, onions, kelp, almonds, tomatoes, carrots, citrus fruits, and red and green peppers.

- Eat foods like citrus fruits, broccoli, carrots, and green leafy veggies. These foods are high in vitamin C, vitamin E, vitamin A, and riboflavin, which are excellent free-radical scavengers. Free radicals and toxins are by-products of stress and environmental pollutants. They are also implicated in aging and disease. Did you know that free radicals cause cars to rust?

- Eat less animal fats, fried foods, and fats that are solid at room temperature. These fats contain more LDL cholesterol. Heart experts have defined LDL cholesterol as "less desirable" because it gums up the lining of blood vessels. HDL cholesterol is desirable because it is transported to the liver where it is either sent out as waste or used in important hormone production. HDL may actually help pick up LDL cholesterol in arteries and clear it from the body. (Immediately following a workout, HDL can be temporarily increased by up to 20%.)

- Invest in one or two sessions with a doctor and/or registered dietician. It may cost $60.00 to $100.00 per visit—although many health-care plans provide coverage. The individualized information can save years of uncertainty about nutritional deficiencies or food allergies.

- Have you ever eaten to the point of having to unbutton your pants? UCLA's Dr. Roy Walford reports that he could extend the lifespan of mice five times by feeding them less food. His research points to the concept that overeating puts a strain on the human body and shortens life. He recommends that you eat to a level of comfort, and put your fork away! Dr. Deepak Chopra also agrees with this concept. His findings suggest eating until the stomach is full taxes your system unnecessarily. Because the stomach is a muscular bag, it is best filled up only to two-thirds and the rest left empty for digestive action. The concept being: the less energy used for digestion could then be used for other functions in the body–mental tasks, physical movement and for repair of injuries.

Philosophers and researchers into the human condition have come to the conclusion that we have control over one thing in life: our attitude. Picture in your mind a 75-year-old couple. What do they look like, and what kind of things would they be doing. What is their posture like, and how healthy are they? Do this now, before you read the next paragraph.

What you have just imagined is indicative of your beliefs about old age. Ultimately, with your present beliefs, this is how you will look at 75. If you did not like your vision, then you must take responsibility now. Beginning to let go of those preconceived notions of what one should look and feel like at a certain age is the first step towards growing older with fascination instead of fear and trepidation.

> **"To see a world in a grain of sand**
> **And heaven in a wild flower,**
> **To hold Infinity**
> **In the palm of your hand,**
> **And Eternity in an hour."**
> **~William Blake**

Part Three:

Creating Balance

"In every aspect of our lives, we are always
asking ourselves:
How am I of value? What is my worth?
Yet I believe that worthiness is our birthright."
~Oprah

CHAPTER THIRTEEN

BODY IMAGE: Mirror, Mirror on the Wall...

> "Self-esteem isn't everything.
> It's just there's nothing without it."
> ~Gloria Steinem

HOW THE WORLD VIEWS US

Of all our senses, sight is the most keenly developed. We begin storing pictures in our minds from the first day we open our eyes as infants. We remember the feelings associated with these images and soon learn the importance of visual appeal in our mass-market culture.

Our first impressions are often based solely on physical appearance. The old adage, "You don't get a second chance to make a first impression" holds true! Sure, people shouldn't judge each other on appearance alone. But, the fact is, people see the outside first and look on the inside later.

The media plays a huge part in how we think we should look as well as how we view others. We are bombarded with countless images of "perfection" on television and in movies. But this is not reality; it is just a representation of the popular culture.

Do you realize how many people have major challenges in the area of body image? No one is immune. Long-legged supermodel Cindy Crawford has been reported as saying she doesn't like her hips. Shania Twain reported she felt her legs were too short and her thighs too big. And the list goes on...

In fact, some of you may be sitting right now in your comfortable home saying, "If only I were ten pounds lighter or two inches taller..." Or, "If only my legs were longer or the back of my arm didn't jiggle when I say goodbye to my friends..."

DID YOU KNOW?

The average woman in North America is a size 12? We seem to have this mass belief that in the ideal world, women should all be a size 2, like Jennifer Aniston on the hit television show *Friends*. Jacqueline Hope, a very special lady, gives hope to the average woman. As the first mainstream plus-sized model, Hope allowed everyday woman to see that they too could be sexy and alluring, even in the high-fashion world.

"Having been on both sides of the physical fence,
I know I prefer being in top shape! Not being physically fit is a heavy
burden to carry through life..."
~Cary C.

As a former athlete who is now more than 110 pounds over my competition weight, I know a thing or two about body image. Indeed, I've been at both physical extremes. About nine years ago, I was in fabulous shape. Having dedicated myself to eating right and working out regularly, I looked and felt great. And people noticed.

I have to admit, I loved the attention, too. I remember once walking into a restaurant with my training partner. Months of weight training and attention to diet had made their mark. On this particular summer evening, four young women about our age were all smiles in a corner of the restaurant as we put in our orders at the counter. They flirted harmlessly. For my friend and me, it was an innocent ego trip. We waved to the girls on our way out, and they waved back.

Presently, at 280 pounds, I am experiencing the other side of the coin. My excess bodyweight has affected almost every aspect of my public and private life. It crosses my mind throughout my day and many times leaves me tired and depressed.

HOW WE SEE OURSELVES

It's extremely difficult for many people to separate their opinion of themselves and their body image. In the September 2000 People Magazine, we read that out of one thousand women surveyed, only 10% were happy with their body! The rest of the women reported feelings of depression or stress about their figures - some had even declined social invitations on occasion because of their discomfort with their weight.

The fact of the matter is - you are not alone. Even the "most beautiful" people on the planet feel inadequate at times. Focus on your attributes and take care of yourself. Make your body the best that it can be!

"I have learned to make the most of what I have and
to celebrate my own positive attributes. "
~Kary

I had the opportunity to listen to Michelle LeMay (fitness celebrity, former sport aerobic competitor) speak at a fitness conference a few years ago in Toronto. She spoke about the decisions people may make because of society's standards. Rarely do we see advertising depicting the inner qualities of people; instead, we're bombarded with the superficial qualities, such as hair, bodyfat, facial beauty, breast size, etc. We all go through periods when we feel inadequate, and often, we find ourselves comparing our physical attributes to those of others.

Many decisions about cosmetic surgeries are based on these comparisons and our ideas about what others want to see. Michelle referred to this as the voice of the ego. When you make a decision based on your ego, you are thinking about what the decision will mean to others. So before you make a decision, it is important to ask yourself what your true self really feels. Listen to your intuition or your inner voice—it always tells the truth. Base your decision on how you really feel and how it will affect your life. Take the time to make this honest assessment of your wants and needs without worrying about how anyone else will react.

When you are making any important long-term cosmetic decision, first educate yourself through reading and talking to experts in the area. Next assess your future goals, plans, and image and decide if it will aid you on your journey. Consider the effect your decisions could have on those who look to you as a role model, e.g., your children. What messages do you want to send them?

"I was brought to believe that how I saw myself
was more important than how others saw me."
~Anwar El-Sadat

IMPRESS YOURSELF!

Most people begin exercise and healthy eating programs for appearance reasons. The road to fitness is rarely chosen because of a desire to feel good. But, that's okay. Do whatever it takes to get you going in the beginning. The key is to get started. At some point, you will realize that there are more reasons to stay fit than the reflection in the bathroom mirror.

We think that people have it backwards in society. We try so hard to impress others that we fail to be impressed with ourselves. If we could learn how to be happy in our own bodies and comfortable with ourselves, then other people's opinions wouldn't matter so much. Often, we're so busy wondering what the other person is thinking, we're missing out on the enjoyment to be had.

20 BODY-IMAGE BOOSTERS

- Focus on what you like most about yourself. Energy flows where your attention goes. Paying more attention to your good attributes (we're sure you can come up with at least one!) will slowly make you feel better. Avoid body-bashing statements like: "my thighs are too big," and replace them with an affirmation like, "I'm grateful to have strong legs that can move my body." Take charge of the degrading self-talk. Get out of the vicious cycle of attacking yourself with your thoughts. Always focusing on parts you don't like can have negative effects on your entire outlook.

DID YOU KNOW?
Constantly entertaining negative thoughts has a tendency
to spill over into your posture, words, and actions.

**"Every person is what he is because of the dominating
thoughts which he permits to occupy his mind."**
~Napolean Hill

- Keep in mind the fact that people are attracted to people who are comfortable with their self-images. There are many telltale signs of a good body image: excellent posture, an easy smile, a confident stride, and maybe even a bounce to the step. These traits have universal appeal in our culture.

**"I like characters who don't feel sorry for themselves.
Self-pity isn't a very sympathetic or seductive trait."**
~Actress Glenn Close

- Take care of what you wear and how you wear it. Wear proper fitting clothes (not necessarily expensive designer names) that are clean and wrinkle free; they enable you to present a better image to the outside world.

- Stop comparing yourself with other people. We are all different shapes and sizes. At any one time, you will either be in better condition or worse condition than the people around you.

> **"Happiness is being able to acknowledge that**
> **you are enough just the way you are right now."**
> **~David Baird**

- Do not participate in endless conversations about diet, food, and body-weight. These discussions rarely end on a positive note. Have you ever noticed that you often leave those conversations feeling drained?

- Stop weighing yourself every day. The scale is the instrument of the chronic dieter who focuses on the numbers rather than the feelings of living a healthy lifestyle. Do not use old clothing as another form of measurement. Our bodies are constantly changing, and it is not fair to yourself to expect the jeans you wore a decade ago to fit perfectly today!

- Acknowledge the fact that public opinion changes like the wind. In the Victorian Age, they admired plumpness. During the Roaring Twenties, thin was in. The fifties championed the hourglass figure. In the sixties, with the fascination of youth culture and freedom, models like Twiggy flourished. Do you want your body image to be dictated by public sentiment? Or, do you want to be in the driver's seat of your own life?

- Start investing in the basics of good health and fitness: such as a good pair of walking shoes, a mountain bike, a health-conscious cooking class, a subscription to informative magazines on lifestyle fitness. Taking action is a great way to move past petty concerns of, "I wonder what they think of me?"

- Avoid the quick fixes. People rationalize using unhealthy techniques (liquid diets, abusing laxatives) to lose weight for a special event. A friend's wedding or a high-school reunion may re-awaken their private body war.

> **"Whenever you find yourself wondering what others are**
> **thinking about you– remember that they are probably**
> **wondering what you are thinking about them!"**
> **~ Kary**

- Motion drives emotion. It's hard to feel depressed when you are moving quickly and breathing deeply. Going for a walk in nature gets the heart beating faster and blood circulating. The next level would be an aerobic workout or resistance training. The very act of exercising creates energy.

- Take care of yourself! Schedule massages or spend an entire day at a spa. By spending time and energy on yourself, you are declaring that *you are valuable!*

- Focus on your true desires and dreams. Actively pursuing them will give you a renewed zest for life.

- Be realistic! How much time and energy do you want to commit to looking a certain way? A body with excellent muscle tone and low bodyfat (e.g., an Olympic gymnast or a ballerina) requires many hours of exercise per day and excellent eating habits.

- Take advantage of the science of positive self-talk. There is documented evidence that what we say to ourselves on a daily basis affects how we feel. We have 50,000 thoughts per day. Experts say 80% of these thoughts are negative or self-limiting. Can you imagine a world-class sprinter at an Olympic final in the 100-meter dash with a negative self-talk? Could you imagine that same athlete verbally abusing himself with disparaging comments under his breath and still winning? A subtle change in your self-talk can and will affect every area of your life.

Just for today, why don't you keep track of how often you put yourself down or criticize yourself?

- Having a new inner vision allows you to face life head on and get more out of life. Living with a sense of purpose gives you the ability to transcend petty worries and needless fears. You will come from an "I deserve it" attitude.

"I think the key to life is being yourself.
I'd rather be Earl Campbell than anyone else...
I don't think it is a good idea to look at somebody else and tell yourself:
'I would like to be just like him.'"
~Earl Campbell (Former NFL star)

THE REAL YOU

Being aware of who you are and what you stand for is very liberating. Essentially, being more aware will lead to expending less energy on distractions. Instead of scattered thoughts, you will begin to have steadiness of mind. You will begin to take more responsibility for your life. That empowering feeling of, "If it is to be, it is up to me" is an important one to cultivate. It has benefits that could affect every aspect of your existence.

You will make fewer excuses for the condition you find yourself in. This will put you in the driver's seat—the person who can make decisions. From this vantage point, you can accurately assess your level of health and fitness. Now you can make health and nutrition decisions and choices based on what your "true self" intuitively knows is right for you.

Our deepest fear is not that we are inadequate;
our deepest fear is that we are powerful beyond measure.
It is our light, not our darkness, that most frightens us.
We ask ourselves, who am I to be brilliant, gorgeous, talented, and
fabulous?
Actually, who are you not to be?
You are a child of God.
Your playing small doesn't serve the world.
There's nothing enlightened about shrinking
so that other people won't feel insecure around you.
We were born to make manifest the glory of God that is within us.
It's not just in some of us, it is in everyone.
And as we let our own light shine,
we unconsciously give other people permission to do the same.
As we are liberated from our own fear,
our presence automatically liberates others.

~Nelson Mandela's Inaugural Speech

Feel the power of the words you have just read and breathe in deeply. Close your eyes and think about how amazing it would be to free yourself from the opinions of others.

"To thine own self be true."
~William Shakespeare

SUGGESTED READING:

Living, Loving, & Learning by Leo Buscaglia, Ph.D.
This is an exquisite collection of the author's lectures and stories. He challenges you to celebrate your inadequacies, choose life, and stop running yourself down. LOVE is the theme that runs throughout the book.

"Don't take yourself too seriously.
And don't be too serious about not taking
yourself too seriously."
~Howard Ogden

CHAPTER FOURTEEN

LAUGH YOUR WAY TO HEALTH
80

> **"Of all the gifts bestowed by nature on human beings,**
> **hearty laughter must be close to the top."**
> **~Norman Cousins**

HUMOUR AS A HEALER

There are numerous studies on the benefits of laughter. William Fry, M.D., author of numerous papers on the benefits of laughter, contended that an extended session of laughter is equivalent to a session of exercise. Stacks of research show there's a connection between laughter and immune-system enhancement. Laughter has also been shown to have a positive impact on the skeletal muscular system, the central nervous system, the respiratory system, the cardiovascular system, and the endocrine system. And it appears to be one of the best natural defences against depression! It's too bad you can't buy it at the drugstore.

> **On the topic of Herbs:**
> **" I take dandelion, passion flower, hibiscus – I feel great.**
> **And when I pee, I experience the fresh scent of potpourri"**
> **~comedian Sheila Wenz**

Should hospitals hire nurses or doctors who have a background in stand-up comedy? That could be a little challenging. Perhaps the most difficult part would be finding the insurance code for the hospital to charge for those services.

> **"There ain't much fun in medicine,**
> **but there's a heck of a lot of medicine in fun."**
> **~Josh Billings**

Dr. Norman Cousins, best-selling author of *Anatomy of an Illness*, had an interesting story. He was a hard-working, popular professor at the school of medicine at UCLA. Later in his career, he was confined to a hospital bed with an aggressive connective-tissue disorder that limited his mobility. It caused extreme inflammation of his joints and spine and put him in great pain.

Dr. Cousins asked a friend to set up a movie screen so he could watch Marx Brother's movies and *Candid Camera* reruns all day. When he found that ten minutes of belly laughter gave him two hours without pain, he knew he was onto something! Even his doctors noticed that their patient not only looked better but also needed a lot less pain medication than they had been giving him. With the positive effects of his own special humour therapy, he eventually recovered most of his mobility.

**"Laughter is so beneficial physically
that it's like inner jogging."
~Norman Cousins**

Wilfred Peterson, author of *The Art of Living*, also recommends laughter as a healing force. He noted that laughter sets healing vibrations into motion and can fill any room with the sunshine of good cheer. Injecting laughter can soothe a tense situation, calm a temper, and undo frazzled nerves. He said a daily prescription of "don't take yourself so damned seriously" would work wonders for all of us.

Laughter not only triggers endorphins, the body's natural painkillers, it also increases the levels of serotonin, one of the hormones connected with our sense of peace and security. **He who laughs… lasts!**

**"I realize that a sense of humour isn't for everyone.
It's only for people who want to have fun, enjoy life,
and feel alive."
~Anne Wilson Schaef**

DID YOU KNOW...

Laughter improves respiration and gently raises pulse and blood pressure before generating a relaxed state. It takes 43 muscles to frown versus only 17 to smile. (This is the only time we'll give you permission to use fewer muscles in an exercise!)

LAUGHING TOGETHER

"Giddy with only two hours of sleep
and the anticipation of another adventure..."
~Kary

We had planned a repeat of our January 1, 1999, fantasy California wedding adventure for the dawn of the new millennium. Even with the implied Y2K doom forecast of Armageddon, we packed our protein powder, camera, and California clothing essentials. Our alarm shrilly announced the arrival of our departure day at 4:00 am December 29, 1999. Giddy with only two hours of sleep and the anticipation of another adventure, we headed off to the airport.

We were a little nervous when the cab driver asked if he could turn the meter off and get paid in cash. He upped the ante when he started casually flashing his headlights on and off at every intersection. Forget about our Y2K worries, we were not even sure we were going to make it to the airport!

Fishtailing and screeching brakes made the ride a little less than comforting. Thoughts of gang violence and images of a James Bond exit from the backseat ripped through our active imaginations. It didn't help when we stopped at an ATM to get some money: Uche exited the cab, and the driver turned to me with an emotionless face and asked: "Is that your husband?"

That five-minute ride to the airport could have been the opening scene to a Michael Crichton movie! We arrived abruptly at the airport, and with silent agreement, gave the guy a handsome tip – after all, he knew where we lived!

Did you know that sharing funny stories and laughter with the important people in your life could strengthen the bond of your relationships? When you regularly laugh with your loved ones (not *at* them!), you begin associating good feelings with their presence.

"Among those whom I like, I can find no common denominator, but among those whom I love, I can: all of them make me laugh."
~W.H. Auden

INCORPORATE LAUGHTER INTO YOUR DAY

The love doctor Leo Buscaglia recommended that adults get in touch with their *kookiness* again. He reports that people take themselves too seriously and that bursts of laughter decrease as we age. He suggests living a little "nutty" occasionally. That alone can brighten any dreary day.

> **"A little nonsense now and then is cherished**
> **by the wisest men."**
> **~Willy Wonka, from *Charlie and the Chocolate Factory***

Our wish for you is a life full of laughter and all of the health and soulful benefits that come with it! Laughter opens your heart and massages the soul. Start massaging today.

> **"The grandest of things are achieved with a light heart:**
> **allow your soul to smile."**
> **~Shirley MacLaine**

HAPPINESS HOMEWORK

- Go to a comedy club or dinner theater with friends or your significant other on a regular basis.

- Go to your local bookstore and browse through the humour section – take a friend if you don't like laughing alone!

- Write down a list of activities that could bring more light and laughter to your life in your journal. Show this list to someone who might want to join you.

- Rent funny movies with some of your most outrageous friends.

- Go to the zoo during mating season. This is guaranteed to bring a smile to your face. Have you ever seen turtles mate?

> **"He who has achieved success, has lived well,**
> **laughed often, and loved much."**
> **~African proverb**

SUGGESTED READING:

Papa, My Father by Leo Buscaglia
An extremely warm book filled with great personal stories from the author's childhood.

"Remember you have an obligation
to yourself to make your life on this earth
as happy as possible."
~Maxwell Maltz

CHAPTER FIFTEEN

CREATING BALANCE IN YOUR LIFE
&

"All work and no play makes Jack a dull boy."
~Anonymous

"It was the perfect time for Uche and I to look inside
ourselves and re-evaluate our schedules..."
~Kary

     We had such full lives when we first got together. I was teaching physical education part time, conducting gymnastics clinics, and competing in fitness contests all over the world. Uche was working full time as a dentist, exercising regularly, and attending professional development seminars all over North America. We knew we needed to take time for reflection and relaxation or, as well-known author Dr. Stephen Covey says, "sharpening the saw."

     We were attending a course called "Soul Psychology" offered by Eileen Montroy, and one night we were racing to make it there on time. Eating in the truck as we drove frantically down the Winnipeg streets, we realized the irony of the situation. I couldn't stop laughing when I looked over and saw Uche writing in his day planner at a red light!

"We are walking on a tightrope,
always living with the threat of falling off.
We seem to lack the one simple ingredient
that would change it all – BALANCE."
~Patricia Raskin, author of *Success, Your Dream and You*

A LIFE SIMPLIFIED?

     Have you noticed the number of people with two career families: their day-planners spilling over; their children running to endless after-school activities; their cell phones, pagers, and laptops accompanying them everywhere? Why does it seem so many people are taking on everything instead of focusing on doing a few things well?

"Do what you can with what you have, where you are."
~Theodore Roosevelt

Have you ever had a time in your life when even the simplest task seemed overwhelming? A time when there just wasn't enough time to get everything done? A time when exhaustion and irritability led to reduced productivity in your life?

The one area that probably suffered the most was your health and fitness. Your nutrition and exercise usually take a backseat to the crises caused by poor management of daily tasks or by simply taking on too much.

"Constantly switching gears was becoming
more and more of a challenge."
~Uche

I remember several years ago going home after a 12-hour day of seeing patients. I was feeling satisfied but exhausted. And it was only Tuesday! I had decided I deserved a break that day and was in line at a drive thru, waiting to place my order. It was the perfect time to call back a few patients from the day to see how they were recovering from their procedures. I was in the process of looking for a phone number as it became my turn to order into the speaker. I almost asked the drive-thru employee how she was doing after her dental extraction. I chuckled and quickly corrected my words.

No one has ever proclaimed on his or her deathbed:
"I wish I would have spent more time at work!"

In Dr. Steven Lamm's book, *Younger at Last: The New World of Vitality Medicine*, he shares that increasing job pressures have placed tremendous strain on many of our lives. He found that optimal stamina, energy, and health were becoming mandatory with high work performance standards, urgent emails, and continuous multi-tasking.

Elaine St. James, the author of *Living the Simple Life*, has written a great guide to scaling down and enjoying more of what really brings you joy. It is so easy to get caught up in "having and doing" in life - that just "being" often gets postponed to that far off place called "Some day I'll…"

Losing that hunger for bigger, newer, and more expensive items opens the door for you to look inside yourself for what really would bring you satisfaction – maybe a supportive relationship with your family and better health. A new sense of freedom can result from this celebration of a new consciousness.

This does not mean you have to sell everything and move your family to a log cabin out in the middle of nowhere. (Although some of us may benefit from that.)

"It is possible to own too much. A man with one watch knows what time it is; a man with two watches is never quite sure."
~Lee Segall

14 BALANCED-LIFE BLOCKERS

- Working extended hours on a regular basis
- Skipping meals
- Taking work with you on your holidays
- Having no health and fitness standards for yourself
- Continually focusing on past emotional hurts and misdeeds
- Lack of communication with significant others
- Not spending time in nature on a regular basis
- Erratic sleep patterns – depriving yourself most days and then playing catch-up on weekends
- Not celebrating any of your successes or accomplishments
- Having unsupportive relationships
- Poor time-management skills
- Not keeping a journal or daily planner
- Addictions

If you found three or more of the above points applying to your life, you're certainly not alone! But it's time to make a mid-course correction on your journey! The exciting thing is that the moment you set a new standard for yourself, you begin to become a new person. It's sometimes hard to believe that one simple degree of change in how you think or behave can alter your destiny. But it's the truth!

"The biggest lie people tell themselves is that self-defeating behaviours aren't going to cost them anything...they do."
~Dr. Mark Goulston

TAKING A TIMEOUT

Having regular timeouts are important to living a fully functioning life. The physical and mental benefits are numerous: better rest and relaxation, a feeling of balance, increased well-being through elevated levels of the brain chemical serotonin, increased immune-system function, and lowered resting heart rate. There is nothing like a little solitude and quiet time to rejuvenate yourself.

"A moment of insight gleaned during
solitude could save years of looking for answers."
~Uche

The advantages of quiet contemplation seem numerous. The challenging part is creating time to do it. I have the best intentions to make it a permanent part of my life. I guess there's a part of me that believes that being busy will bring me results faster. However, from everything I have read and experienced, a moment of insight gleaned during some solitude could save years of looking for answers. The decision appears simple, doesn't it? Well, let's see how I do today...

Looking back or reflecting can be a great investment in your future. You can gather the lessons from your past and invest them in your next year. So instead of living each year flying by the seat of your pants, you can move with more elegance and certainty into the future. As a result, you may become a better mother, a better father, a better spouse, a better friend, a better worker, or a better athlete.

Try spending a few minutes each day looking back on the various lessons you've learned. We use a special room in our home that's lined with hundreds of books we have collected over the years. It's painted a very soothing lilac colour. There are African masks and incense holders decorating the walls. When the window is open in the early morning, we can hear nature's melody outside telling us we're alive and well. Every time we step into its sanctuary, we feel relaxed.

Do you have a place in your home where you feel a sense of peace and serenity? Could you set aside a space in your home where you could have a special sanctuary?

WORK CAN ENHANCE YOUR LIFE

> **"To love what you do and know that it matters—**
> **what could be more fun?"**
> **~Katherine Graham**

In the bestseller by Marsha Sinetar, *Do What You Love and the Money Will Follow*, she reported that working in an area that you are passionate about is fulfilling and good for your health. Ask yourself the following questions and take some time to reflect on your answers:

1.   What are your feelings as you go to work each morning?

2.   When you are asked what you enjoy doing, do you mention your job?

3.   Do you ever experience frequent stomach upset, heart palpitations, headaches, or backaches?

4.   Would you say you're in the best shape of your life right now?

5.   Would you say you're just trying to get through the week?

6.   Are you engaging in any self-destructive behaviour?

7.   Do you find yourself thinking about work when you are with your family and thinking about your family when you're at work—with neither getting your full attention?

8.   Would you encourage your children to follow the career path you have chosen?

9.   Would you choose your current career if you had a chance to choose all over again?

"Money—like health, love, happiness, and all forms of miraculous
happenings that you want to create for yourself—
is the result of your living purposefully.
It is not a goal unto itself.
If you chase after it, it will always elude you."
~Dr. Wayne Dyer

OUR TWELVE-POINT TUNE-UP

Have you ever met someone who just seemed to "have it all together"? Smiling often, enjoying and valuing their work, they have a long-term vision and rarely complain about trivial concerns. They make time for family, friends, fitness, and relaxation; and their actions are congruent with their values. They understand that hatred, fear, and jealousy create inner turmoil.

Can you imagine doing what you need to do when it needs to be done according to the standards you have set for yourself? Try incorporating the suggestions below into your day and see if you start seeing a happier, more balanced person smiling back at you in the mirror.

- Exercise regularly. Exercise shapes the mind as well as the body. Adding a fitness regimen allows you to enjoy the endorphins released and an entire range of benefits.

*"I knew it was time to move away from this pain, and
exercise seemed like the best prescription for my woes."
~Kary*

In my early 20's, I started an exercise program because I was fed up with the way I looked and the way I felt. My lifestyle was nowhere near what I had dreamed about as a child and teenager. I was caught up in the throes of self-pity—my boyfriend had just broken up with me, and I felt totally worthless. I had acquired a ton of knowledge about physical fitness in the Faculty of Physical Education, and I wanted to start putting it into action! I began a program that included a little bit of weight training and a lot of cardiovascular activities. Within two weeks, I felt better—not completely healed or euphoric, but I knew I was doing something good for myself, and my wounds slowly started to heal. Three years later, fitness had become something I did for my own pleasure. Working out brought balance to my life. To this day, exercise is an immediate elixir for me!

- Include deep breathing, meditation, or yoga in your daily activities. One of the most rejuvenating practices is the art of sitting alone, detached from your daily tasks. The energy gained and the insights gleaned are beyond belief.

- Practice forgiveness. It is a simple tool that may lighten your psychological load.

- Learn to say "NO." Attempting to please everyone leads to feeling overwhelmed and frustrated. It's a sure fire way to take the balance out of your life.

- Set goals in every area of your life: family, financial, health, social, intellectual, and spiritual. Review these goals weekly (include your family) and have concrete, measurable ways of assessing their achievement. Remember you are the CEO of You, Inc.

- Learn to laugh more at life's absurdities and be able to share them with the special people in your life.

- Make better nutrition choices (remember our tips from chapter 7 - Food for Function) and find ways to stick to your resolve.

- Take vacation time and actually use it to simply enjoy your time off. Leave your laptop, pager, electronic organizer, and cell phone at home!

"Life is not a stress rehearsal."
~Loretta LaRoche

- Do your best in all that you do. Going after perfection means you will never be satisfied with any result you get. This type of standard leads to frustration, anxiety, and anger. Aim for excellence instead of perfection.

- Enjoy living in the moment more often. Have you ever been so immersed in something that you lost track of time? Spending more time in the present means you will worry less about the past and the future.

- Try colour breathing! It has been reported by Chinese healers that visualizing the colours of the spectrum can help relax you and bring you peace. Research has shown that colour affects you emotionally and physically. Chinese colour therapists say that by first taking a deep breath and clearing your mind, you can imagine breathing in a colour and let it flood your body. For example, breathing in the colour green – the colour of nature – may stimulate that part of the nervous system that relaxes the muscle in your chest and help you breathe more slowly.

- Read about topics that interest you. There is nothing like losing yourself in a good book to lighten life's load. Books allow the curious person to tap the treasure chest of others' experiences. If you don't know where to start looking, just head down to your local bookstore and browse.

"What helps keep me balanced is watching for moments when I
can be reminded of what's important."
~Uche

Treating patients in a full time dental practice can be all encompassing. What helps keep me balanced is watching for moments when I can be reminded of what's important. One of the gifts of dealing with people on a daily basis is that I have many opportunities to accomplish this.

One day I was working in my dental office when I was reminded of how fragile life can be. In the middle of a patient's check-up, I realized there was a person waiting in the hallway. It was my patient's husband. He was a doctor who used to fly up to remote northern communities with me. He was in a horrific plane crash in one of those remote towns. Due to the extent of his injuries, he has been left unable to practice and now spends his days in a wheelchair.

Seeing her unquestionable caring and consideration of her husband is incredible. Seeing them interact, I know there's nothing on earth like unconditional love that can sustain and enrich life.

"Don't evaluate your life in terms of achievements…
Instead, wake up and appreciate everything you encounter along the path. Enjoy the flowers that are there for your pleasure. Tune in to the sunrise, the little children, the laughter, the rain, and the birds. Drink it all in… there is no way to happiness; happiness is the way."
~Dr. Wayne W. Dyer, from *Real Magic*

JOURNAL ACTIVITY

Is there an area of your life that you need to simplify?

Identify the times in your week when you feel unbalanced.

What action can you take right now to better care for yourself?

"The human journey involves not just a spiritual awakening but the development of all levels of our being—spiritual, mental, emotional, and physical—and the integration of all these aspects into a healthy and balanced daily life."
~Shakti Gawain, from *Living in the Light*.

SUGGESTED READING:

Living in the Light by Shakti Gawain
This is an excellent read for anyone on a journey of self-discovery.

"Capture the moment, whoever you are.
None of us is here forever."
~Adrian

CHAPTER SIXTEEN

SPIRITUAL FITNESS
ဢ

"We are not human beings with occasional spiritual experiences but
spiritual beings
with occasional human experiences."
~Deepak Chopra

SOMETHING MORE...

Have you ever thought that there was more to you than your body? That there's a part of you that is unchanging and is the true essence of who you are? There is more to becoming healthy and fit then just having a flat stomach. There is spiritual fitness. It refers to the level of harmony between body, mind, and spirit. Wayne Dyer, in *Your Sacred Self*, explains that we grow up believing we are a body, a job, or a nationality. We encourage you to break free from these physical descriptions.

It's an established scientific fact that every seven years, the cells in your body will have been replaced with new cells. This means your physical self is constantly changing and renewing. In other words, eight years ago, your body was comprised of totally different cells than it is today! What part of you is responsible for the memories and feelings from eight or more years ago? The essence of what makes you an individual is beyond the physical – it is timeless, ageless, and without form.

THE RUT AND THE WAY OUT

Often, when people think about fitness, they conjure up images of sweating, sacrifice, and an intense daily effort. They complain about the cost of a gym membership, time spent away from home, and their lack of energy after a long day at work. Fitness is rarely woven into the fabric of life; it is seen as a separate entity. Few people go on to experience the exhilaration of a consistent, long-term commitment to fitness

"I began to look at training for its ability to dissipate stress from my day and to make me feel great. "
~Uche

I had been very busy developing my dental practice and had slowly allowed myself to physically run down. With long 12-hour clinic days working 6 days a week, I was putting my work first and myself second. I would go to a drive-thru restaurant five to six times a week for a fast-food recharge, and I was exercising less and less. My weight was slowly creeping up, and coffee and espressos were my favourite way of recharging my sluggish system.

It was May of 1998, and I was at a three-day conference in California. I decided to give the hotel gym a try during a lunch break. With my gym gear and my good intentions, I headed towards a multi-station weight-training set up. I confidently eased myself into one of the stations and began to exercise– after all, I was a former competitive bodybuilder.

A young guy came over to ask me if I needed a hand. I immediately assumed that he had been impressed with the pace of my workout and wanted to give me a spot (a weight-training term for helping someone with the last few repetitions of a challenging set).

No, he replied, I just wanted to know if you needed some instructions with the machines. I was confused – couldn't he tell I was an expert in weight training? I looked sideways into a mirror and suddenly realized it was a different figure staring back. It certainly wasn't the toned, fit figure of my college days, ten years ago.

I let him proceed with his goodwill gesture and in that moment made a commitment to reclaim my health and fitness. After the conference, I continued making all kinds of changes in my living habits. Sure I had some times when I slid backwards. But, I did not beat myself up over it. I would get back on track and make more improvements.

I began to look at exercising for its ability to dissipate stress from my hectic days and to make me feel great. Every aspect of my life began to change.

"When you feel good about yourself,
others will feel good about you, too."
~Jake ("Body by Jake") Seinfeld

It is a familiar dilemma. Out of balance— stuck in a rut but continuing to find excuses for not changing the habits that got you there. You intuitively know that taking care of your physical self will benefit every aspect of your life, but you continue to procrastinate. Until you get sick and tired of being "sick and tired," a downward spiral will continue.

Taking that first step on your journey to physical fitness can lead to multiple destinations. Once you have moved passed the "struggle" phase of making fitness a habit, the opportunity for benefits in an entirely different arena is possible. There is the opportunity to achieve something greater from training than just "the burn" after a good workout!

You exercise your psyche as well as your body whenever you partake in physical fitness. It is impossible to work on your body without eventually affecting all of the other areas in your life.

> **"Training gives us an outlet for suppressed energies**
> **created by stress and thus tones the spirit**
> **just as exercise conditions the body."**
> **~Arnold Schwarzenegger**

EXERCISE AS A PATH

In *Working Out, Working Within*, Lynch and Huang reveal that there is increased creativity and mental clarity with the "stillness in motion" achieved during exercise. Because exercise needs such intense focus and concentration, you have the opportunity to transcend your day-to-day challenges. Some people call this "the zone."

So, if you're challenged by something in your life, one of the best ways to get a handle on it is to get moving and enjoy some physical exertion. Through exercising, you may access a wellspring of knowledge and inner creativity. Even going for a short walk can give you a chance to shed some light on a problem. It might be the one thing you haven't done to solve that ongoing personal challenge.

> **"If you do not get it from yourself, where will you go for it?"**
> **~Zenrin, from *The Gospel According to Zen***

"Exercising is meditation for me."
~Kary

Discovering fitness was a major turning point in my life. I began by walking and jogging around the University track. I could not run more than one lap around the track without losing my breath! This soon changed. Every week, I would add one more lap until I finally ran a mile without stopping! This accomplishment gave me the motivation to continue, and I eventually built up to running in a half marathon. I soon took up weight training, and this combined with the cardiovascular activity helped me burn off 18 pounds in about 10 months.

I felt better than ever before, and my self-esteem grew with each new milestone. I saw a dietician and changed some of my eating habits, which led to many positive lifestyle changes. I slowly began to entertain the idea that I could be an athlete, and I started competing in the sport of bodybuilding and fitness.

Every cardio session became time to think about my life and what I wanted to do with it. I found it extremely easy to think like a champion when I was engaged in physical activity. I planned my future during those early workouts, and I have turned most of my dreams into reality.

I connected with my true self during this time and feel closer to God than ever before in my life. I now use my exercise knowledge to help others achieve their goals, and every time I give of myself, I know I have found my true passion in life.

"We do not have a soul. We are a soul that has a body, with functions, needs, and feelings. We have a body to experience, and we gain experience for the soul."
~Shirley Maclaine,
from *Going Within: a Guide for Inner Transformation*

MEDITATION: A PATHWAY TO SPIRITUAL FITNESS

"Mother, knows best..."
~Uche

I graduated from University with a wealth of technical and clinical information. I could do extremely challenging dental procedures and recite facts to back up any point of view. I was able to work a full ten-hour day and go to the gym- without a break. I felt invincible at the age of 28.

One day my brother, Chiedu, gave me a video called Live Your Dreams with inspirational speaker Les Brown. I became fascinated with the topic of what made human beings tick. I began to take workshops in my city. I became adventurous and invested in conferences outside my city (and later the country). I had the opportunity to meet and learn from some amazing people at the forefront of personal development and spirituality.

I enrolled in courses on meditation, self-development, and communication. The list was endless.

I felt I was really beginning to get a grasp on the entire subject. But, it always brings a smile to my face when I remember a telephone conversation with my mother – I was trying to explain some challenge I was facing. I told her I was about to try one of the new strategies I had learned at an expensive three-day, professional lecture series. She replied, "Have you tried praying yet?

Jon Kabat-Zinn's book, *Wherever You Go, There You Are,* defines meditation as a way of being, living, and listening – a way of being in harmony with things as they are. Enjoying a reflective component in our daily lives may be essential to happiness and peace of mind, but how many of us are making time for it? Perhaps we should take the hint from Ricky Martin, Oprah Winfrey, Madonna, and John Travolta – just a few well-known people who have acknowledged that an inner journey is essential to success.

**"If your mind isn't clouded by unnecessary things,
this is the best season of your life."
~Wu-Men**

Many people have the misconception that the only way to meditate is to sit in the lotus position with a candle. But there are numerous meditative strategies stemming from different religions and philosophies. Meditation doesn't have to be a complicated process. It can be as simple as closing your eyes and taking some deep breaths before you leave for work. It can be as simple as enjoying the sound of water falling over rocks or the air passing through your nostrils into your lungs. Your mind has a sense of clarity, of being free from the stress of self-consciousness. Time is unimportant and seems to fly by. These are moments when you are carefree and joyful; these are moments of flow that can occur anytime, anywhere.

**"The only journey worth taking is the journey within."
~Yeats**

TRY THIS:
The next time you are feeling a little down, take a time out and turn inward. Instead of turning on the television, reading a magazine, or going to the refrigerator, get comfortable in a chair or on the floor. Just sit down and take some deep breaths, if only for a minute or two. Simply sit and be still. See if you are able to recapture some energy.

You will be in good company if you start the practice of meditation: spiritual sages throughout history have spent a part of their day in silence or meditation. This regular discipline added to your schedule would provide an opportunity for you to review your day and make daily adjustments for tomorrow. Denying yourself time for your soulful, boundless, spiritual side would be like a lumberjack chopping down trees, day after day, without ever sharpening his axe.

We've read that 4:00 am is a great time to awaken and be alone with your thoughts. Spiritual teachers throughout the ages have heralded this time of day as a magical time to tap into their consciousness. It is a special time when we're not bothered by distractions, like the telephone or the noise of traffic. Obviously it would take a fair amount of discipline to begin with this practice. So, maybe start with a few minutes of reflection upon rising in the morning.

DID YOU KNOW?
Gandhi and Nelson Mandela resolved many of their inner conflicts when they had isolation thrust upon them in the solitary confinement of prison? It was said that they felt it was the most important time of their lives.

SACRED SPACES

A special spot reserved just for your spiritual fitness may seem like a luxury but is well worth creating. Thomas Edison and Benjamin Franklin had an area set aside in their homes where they sat alone with their thoughts.

Your spot could be located outside if you prefer. Dr. Deepak Chopra loves the idea of a natural sanctuary. He reports that it can increase your prana or chi (life force energy), which has the effect of replenishing or rejuvenating a tired spirit.

This personal time leads to greater self-knowledge and personal power. It allows you to literally tune into infinite wisdom or infinite intelligence or as, Maxwell Maltz, says, "the super conscious". Shirley Maclaine, in her New York Times' best seller *The Camino, a Journey of the Spirit*, reported, "All of life is a lesson in self-knowledge. The more knowledge we have of ourselves, the more we are able to deal with anything."

There's power in silence. Without the silence between the notes, there would be no music! Silent contemplation can and will deliver many gifts for you. Not only will it make you stronger mentally and spiritually, it will have surprising effects on you physically.

**"Learn to get in touch with silence within yourself and know that everything in this life has a purpose.
There are no mistakes, no coincidences.
All events are blessings given to us to learn from."
~Elisabeth Kübler-Ross, M.D.**

THE ART OF RELAXATION

Wilfred Peterson was a writer who was known for practicing what he preached about joyful living. He lived to a ripe 94 years of age, and his bestseller *The Art of Living* was the culmination of a lifetime of growth and learning. He suggests that people must learn to shatter the stresses of daily living, or the stresses will shatter them. We must learn to bend like a willow tree with life's strains and stresses, and by doing so, spring back after the storms of life have passed.

Dr. Melvyn Kinder, in *Going Nowhere Fast*, reaffirms how finding peace of mind can be achieved by stepping off of life's treadmill periodically. Our desire for the ideal career, the perfect mate, the body beautiful, and picture-perfect children can be all-consuming. People can become so busy trying to maintain the life they thought they wanted. Then one day, they're not so certain. And they realize they have forgotten about true enjoyment.

Many people who lead crazy, fast-paced lives say they are too busy to sit still. "I'm busy, busy, busy." They almost brag about not having time to relax. In our modern world, it is very easy to become consumed with one project after another when climbing the ladder of success. One day you may realize your ladder is against the wrong wall, and you are standing on the top rung all alone.

> **"Slow down and take the time to really see.**
> **Take a moment to see what is going on**
> **around you right now, where you are. You may be missing**
> **something wonderful."**
> **~J. Michael Thomas**

ALTER YOUR PHYSICAL REALITY

By working on yourself to achieve inner harmony, you can alter your physical reality. Every one of the 100 trillion cells in our bodies is affected by our thoughts and feelings. Each of those cells is eavesdropping on our inner and outer dialogue. Unless we acknowledge this connection, we can find ourselves caught up in a spiral of aches, pains, and medications. To begin healing, we must first take responsibility for the condition we are in. If we are at the top of the list for causes of the pain, then we can be at the top of the list for solutions.

Louise Hay, metaphysical lecturer and best-selling author of over 20 books, is a strong believer in the power of listening to our body for healing. She says that if we take the time to be silent and to look inward, we would be able to truly listen to what our bodies were saying. In *You Can Heal Your Life,* she explains how the different physical ailments that plague us are mostly caused by toxic thoughts and emotions.

> "What lies behind us and what lies before us
> are tiny matters compared to what lies within us."
> ~Ralph Waldo Emerson

OUR NINE-PART SPIRITUAL PRESCRIPTION

(Try one a day and call us in the morning!)

1. **Spend some time in nature.**

    This could mean taking yourself and your loved ones on a day trip into nature. For example, hiking on a mountain trail, a picnic on an isolated beach, or a trip to the lake. Away from the incessant demands of work and the city, you have the opportunity to get in touch with yourself. There's nothing more refreshing than breathing fresh air and marvelling at the beauty of nature in all her glory!

> "I follow nature as the ultimate guide,
> and resign myself with implicit obedience
> to her sacred ordinances."
> ~Cicero

We were both moved when we read James Redfield's book *Celestine Vision: Living the New Spiritual Awareness*. He writes of special spots and mystical sites on the planet – The Great Pyramids, Stonehenge, and many others. You can visit these places or find your own special spots that give you a sense of well-being, rejuvenation, and energy.

In ancient times, spending time in the sun was thought to connect us with our souls. People would worship the sun for all the gifts it brought them. (Back then they were not as concerned about UV rays.)

> "When I admire the wonder of a sunset
> or the beauty of the moon,
> my soul expands in worship of the Creator."
> ~Mahatma Gandhi

2. **Take a yoga class alone or with a loved one.**

    The Oxford dictionary defines yoga as the Hindu system of physical exercises and breathing control. It is practised to bring one closer with the Universal Spirit. Sounds pretty deep, but, guess what? If your personal fitness and relationships have reached a plateau, this may be the missing link to a whole new level of enjoyment!

> *"We left the yoga studio at an entirely*
> *different pace and peacefully drove home.*
> *What a way to begin a weekend!"*
> *~Kary and Uche*

We made a decision to start learning yoga in January of 2001. Our first class was at 6:30 pm on a Friday evening. After work, we raced to the gym for a weight training session; back home for dinner and a shower, then tore out the door to the yoga studio five miles away. We rushed in and barely had time to grab a space before the instruction started. After an hour and a half of deep-breathing and slow movements, we felt more at peace and rejuvenated.

3. **Try a martial arts course.**
   Many people are drawn to Karate, Kung Fu, and Judo for self-defence but end up realizing there are other benefits. Physical fitness, through the practice of martial arts, can bring tolerance, harmony, and peace of mind.

We condition ourselves to be in charge of our will anytime we follow through with a discipline. This is the definition of willpower. And it can be strengthened like any muscle. We challenge you to give it a workout and enjoy all the benefits.

4. **Practice deep breathing.**
   In Dr. Robert C. Fulford's book *Touch of Life*, he reports that life is defined by breath. The first breath is taken as you enter the world, and the final is taken as you exit. It is our very connection to this world. We have the conscious capacity to take in oxygen and maximize its life force energy. This is an important fact and is integral to being a greater spiritual force on the planet.
   Did you know that when you're angry or scared, you have a tendency to breathe in a shallow manner? To change a state of anger or fear, you only have to begin taking some deep, slow breaths. It will gradually lessen the intensity of the emotion.

"Mankind is not fed by bread alone but also by breath."
~Dr. Robert C. Fulford

5. **Spend some time in an art gallery or museum.**
   The appreciation of art can momentarily assist you in transcending daily challenges. Throughout history art has had a role in raising consciousness. In the Golden Age of Greece, it was statues. Before the Renaissance, suppressed scholars in Europe sought intellectual and spiritual rejuvenation through painting. When could you make time to visit a gallery and tap into this energy? You may not be able to get to Paris today, but every major city and many smaller towns have an art gallery or museum.

6. **Read stimulating books.**
Whenever you feed your mind, you have the opportunity to nourish your spirit. Choose whatever topic turns your crank!

7. **Spend a day at the spa.**
Caring for your physical self will benefit your inner self. If an entire day at a day spa is out of the question, then just book an hour massage – the human touch has healing powers.

8. **Listen to music.**
Have some instrumental CD's close at hand. Try any of Enya's music or Kenny G's beautiful instrumentals for starters. Soothing music can calm frazzled nerves at the end of a long day – especially if you get stuck in traffic on the way home from work.

9. **Look for the gift.**
There is always an equivalent benefit anytime you have a setback in your life. It may not become clear until many years later, but looking for the gift sooner will make your journey through life easier. For example, a man once lost his job. Instead of wallowing in self-pity, he saw his new free time as a gift. He joined a running club while searching for a new job. He met someone at the club who had an excellent business opportunity for him! His choice to make the most of his situation led to many payoffs: his physical health improved, he avoided depression, and he found a new job opportunity.

Writer Henley wrote that we could become the masters of our fates and the captains of our souls. By actually designing our responses, we can be the architects of our destinies! Do not wish for less challenges; ask instead for more strength to handle the obstacles. The gift lies in who you will become when you take on the challenge – head on!

Some of the biggest successes in fitness history have taken place when someone had a crisis in their lives, and their health was challenged. We have seen people become cholesterol experts and "fibre" champions after a life-threatening coronary blockage was diagnosed. We have seen those same people become teachers and role models to others in their community.

"For everything you have missed,
you have gained something else."
~Ralph Waldo Emerson

OUR WISH FOR YOU!

Making a few small, positive changes in your daily habits or your approach to life can have an incredible effect on the mind, body, and soul. More energy, enthusiasm, vitality, love, peak moments, and inner peace are just some of the many gifts you will give yourself.

> **"Can you imagine living one complete day**
> **without thinking about yourself?**
> **Nothing offending you, nothing disturbing you,**
> **nothing causing you to be angry?**
> **Would you then be able to help others?**
> **~Dr. Wayne Dyer**

JOURNAL ACTIVITY

Do you have any people in your life that you would say are spiritually fit?

What spiritual fitness practices do you have in your life?

Which of the Spiritual Prescriptions would you be able to try in the next week?

SUGGESTED READING:

Wherever You Go There You Are by Jon Kabat-Zinn.
This is a very simple and practical guide for anyone to start the practise of meditation.

The Camino by Shirley Maclaine.
Shirley tells of her 500-mile trek through Northern Spain. This is a true story of an intense physical and spiritual challenge.

"This is the true joy in life—being used for a purpose recognized by yourself as a mighty one. Being a force of nature instead of a feverish, selfish little clod of ailments and grievances complaining that the world will not devote itself to making you happy. I am of the opinion that my life belongs to the whole community and as I live, it is my privilege to do for it whatever I can. I want to be thoroughly used up when I die, for the harder I work, the more I love. I rejoice in life for its own sake. Life is no brief candle to me; it is a sort of splendid torch which I've got a hold of for the moment and I want to make it burn as brightly as possible before handing it on to future generations."

~George Bernard Shaw

THE LAST WORD

&

AN INVITATION

Two years ago we started this project out of a desire to help people make fitness a permanent part of their lives. Making fitness a lifelong habit is not possible without powerful reasons. We have written this book to help you uncover your reasons and take immediate action. We hope within these pages you have found strategies and inspiration to make it happen! Enjoying the whole process is the key.

We would love to hear about your journey to fitness. Whether you have overcome an obstacle, surpassed some personal goal, or recovered from an injury or illness, we INVITE you to send us your story. Please include any nutrition or exercise strategies that you used.

Any material submitted becomes the sole property of U.K.O. Enterprises and may be included in an upcoming book.

Please send us your story by email: or regular mail:

U.K.O. Enterprises
Suite 234
162-2025 Corydon Ave.
Winnipeg, Mb.,
Canada R3P 0N5

BIBLIOGRAPHY

Anderson, Dr. James W. & Breecher, Dr. Maury M., *Dr.*
    Anderson's Antioxidant, Antiaging Health Program, Carroll & Graf, 1996
Anthony, Robert, *Doing What You Love, Loving What You Do*, Berkley
    Publishing Group, 1991
Augustine, Sue, *With Wings There Are No Barriers*, Pelican Publishing Company,
    1996
Birch, L.L., Johnson, S.L., Andresen, G., Peters, J.C., and Schulte, M.C.
    The variability of young children's energy intake. *New England Journal*
    of Medicine 324 (1991):232.
Buscaglia, Leo, *Born For Love,* SLACK Incorporated, 1992
Buscaglia, Leo, *Living, Loving, & Learning*, Ballantine Books, 1982
Coehlo, Paulo, *The Alchemist*, HarperCollins, 1993
Chopra, Dr. Deepak, *Magical Mind, Magical Body*, Nightingale-Conant
    Corporation, 1990
Chopra, Dr. Deepak, *Seven Spiritual Laws of Success*,
    Amber-Allen Publishing, 1995
Cousins, Dr. Norman, *Anatomy of An Illness*, Bantam
    Doubleday Dell Publishing, 1991
Cousins, Dr. Norman, *Head First: The Biology of Hope*, Penguin Books, 1989
Covey, Steven, & Covey, Sandra Merrill, *Seven Habits of Highly Effective*
    Families, Golden Books, 1990
Covey, Steven, *Seven Habits of Highly Effective People*, Simon & Schuster, 1989
Covey, Stephen, *The Quest*, Simon & Schuster, 1996
Craig, Jenny, *Jenny Craig's Little Survival Guide*, Leisure Arts, 1996
Crenshaw, L., *The Alchemy of Love and Lust*, Pocket Books, 1997
D'Adamo, Dr. Peter J., Cook Right 4 Your Type, Berkley Books, 1999
Dass, Ram, *Journey of Awakening*, Bantam Books, 1990
Dollemore, Doug, & Giuliucci, Mark, *Age Erasers for Men*, St.
    Martin's Press, 1997
Dyer, Dr. Wayne, Manifest Your Destiny, Nightingale Conant, 1996
Dyer, Dr. Wayne, *Real Magic*, Harper Mass Market
    Paperbacks, 1993
Dyer, Dr. Wayne, *Your Sacred Self*, Harper Collins, 1995
Fletcher, Anne M, *Thin For Life*, Chapters Publishing Ltd., 1994
Fulford, Dr. Robert C., *Dr. Fulford's Touch of Life,* Pocket Books, 1997
Gawain, Shakti, *Living in The Light*, Nataraj Publishing, 1998
Godek, Greg, *Love – The Course They Forgot to Teach you in School*,
    Casablanca Press, 1997
Hakala, Dee, *Thin Is Just A Four Letter Word*, Little, Brown and Company, 1997
Hay, Louise, *You Can Heal Your Life*, Hay House, 1999
Henner, Marilu, *Marilu Henner's Total Health Makeover*, Harper Audio, 1998
Hill, Howard E., *Energizing the 12 Powers of the Mind*, Leisure Books, 1970
Holtz, Lou, *Winning Every Day*, HarperCollins, 1998
Kabat-Zinn, Jon, *Wherever You Go There You Are*, Hyperion, 1994
Kinder, Dr. Melvin, *Going Nowhere Fast*, Fawcett Books, 1991
King, Brad J., *Fat Wars*, Macmillan Canada, 2000
Kirschmann, John D., and Dunne, Lavon J., *Nutrition*
    Almanac – Family Medical and Health Guide, McGraw-Hill, 1998

Lamm, Dr. Steven, *Younger at Last*, Simon & Schuster, 1997

Maclaine, Shirley, *Going Within*, Bantam Doubleday Dell Publishing, 1989

Maclaine, Shirley, *The Camino*, Pocket Books, 2000

Maltz, Maxwell, *Psycho Cybernetics*, Prentice-Hall, 1960

Monaghan, *Why Not Me?,* Prime Books Inc., 1992

Naisbitt, John, and Aburdene, Patricia, *Megatrends 2000*, Avon Books, 1990

Patchell-Evans, David, *Living the Good Life*, Stoddard, 2000

Pearsall, Paul (Ph.D.), *Making Miracles*, Prentice Hall Press, 1991

Pearsall, Paul, *Ten Laws of Lasting Love*, Simon & Schuster, 1993

Perls, Dr. Thomas T., & Silver, Margery, H., *Living To 100: Lessons in Living to Your Maximum Potential at Any Age, Basic Books, 2000*

Peterson, Wilfred, *The Art of Living*, Avon Books, 1990

Philbin, Regis, *I'm Only One Man*, Wheeler Publishing, 1996

Phillips, Bill, *Body For Life*, Harper Collins, 1999

Popcorn, Faith & Marigold, Lys, *Clicking – 16 Trends to Future Fit Your Life, Your Work, and Your Business,* HarperCollins, 1996

Powter, Susan, *Food*, Simon & Schuster, 1995

Pribrim, *Million Dollar Habits*, Crest, 1991

Raskin, Patricia, *Success, Your Dream and You*, Roundtable Publishing, 1991

Redfield, James, *Celestine Prophecy*, Warner Books, 1993

Redfield, James, *Celestine Vision*, Warner Books, 1999

Ringer, Robert, *Million Dollar Habits*, Wynwood Press, 1990

Rippe, Dr. James M., *Fit for Success*, Prentice Hall, 1989

Robbins, Anthony, *Awaken the Giant Within*, Simon and Schuster, 1991

Roger, John and McWilliams, Peter, *Wealth 101*, Prelude Press, 1992

Ruiz, Don M., *The Four Agreements*, Amber-Allen Publishing, 1997

St. James, Elaine, *Living the Simple Life,* Hyperion, 1996

Schwartz, David J., *The Magic of Thinking Big*, Prentice-Hall, 1965

Sharma, Robin S., *The Monk Who Sold His Ferrari*, HarperCollins, 1997

Shubentsov, Yefim, *Cure Your Cravings*,G.P. Putnam's Sons, 1998

Sinetar, Marsha, *Do What You Love and the Money Will Follow*, Dell Publishing, 1987

Somer, Elizabeth, *Food and Mood, Owl Books, 1999* Stewart, Meiji, *Happiness is an Inside Job*, Puddledancer Press, 1997

Thorne & Embleton, *BODYFitness For Women*, Musclemag International, 1999

Timberlake Lewis, *Born to Win*, Tyndale House, 1986

Tribole, Evelyn and Resch, Elyse, *Intuitive Eating– A Recovery Book for the Chronic Dieter,* St. Martin's Press, 1995

Waitley, Dennis, *The Double Win*, Berkley Publishing Group, 1986

Waldman, Mark R., *The Art of Staying Together*, J.P. Tarcher, 1998

Ziglar, Zig, *Over The Top,* Thomas Nelson Publishers, 1994

"You will find, as you look back upon your life, that the moments that stand out are the moments when you have done things for others."
~Henry Drummond

This book would make the perfect gift!

Order a signed copy of *Fit for the LOVE of It!*

Web orders: www.fitlove.com
Mail orders: send check or money order to:

U.K.O. Enterprises
Suite 234
162-2025 Corydon Avenue
Winnipeg, Manitoba
Canada R3P 0N5
E-mail: fitlove@shaw.ca

Please send me __ copy(s) of Fit For the Love of It at
$19.95 CANADIAN or $13.95 US each, plus applicable taxes.

Please add $3.00 per book for shipping and handling.
(Out of North America, priority request, or bulk orders - please call for price quote.)

Cheque/ Money Order enclosed for $ _____
(Payable to: U.K.O. Enterprises)

OR

Charge my: _____Visa

Account #:_____ Expiry Date:_____

Signature:_____Print Name:_____

Send my signed copy to:

Address:_____

City: _____Province/State:_____

Country:_____Postal Code:_____

Telephone:_____E-mail:_____

NOTES